D0436623

JUN   2008

FORENSICS

and

FICTION

Also by D. P. Lyle, M.D.

Murder and Mayhem
Forensics for Dummies

Thomas Dunne Books / St. Martin's Minotaur New York

FORENSICS

and

FICTION

*Clever, Intriguing, and Downright Odd
Questions from Crime Writers*

D. P. Lyle, M.D.

THOMAS DUNNE BOOKS.
An imprint of St. Martin's Press.

www.thomasdunnebooks.com
www.minotaurbooks.com

Library of Congress Cataloging-in-Publication Data

Lyle, D. P.
Forensics and fiction : clever, intriguing, and downright odd questions from crime writers / D. P. Lyle.—1st ed.
    p.   cm.
  ISBN-13: 978-0-312-36551-6
  ISBN-10: 0-312-36551-9
1. Detective and mystery stories—Miscellanea. 2. Forensic sciences—Miscellanea.

PN3448.D4 L93 2007
809.3'872—dc22   2007013794

First Edition: August 2007

10 9 8 7 6 5 4 3 2 1

THIS BOOK IS TO PROVIDE WRITERS OF FICTION WITH ANSWERS TO BASIC AND COMPLEX QUESTIONS ON MED-ICAL AND FORENSIC ISSUES. IT IS NOT TO BE USED FOR DIAGNOSIS OR FOR REAL-LIFE BEHAVIOR.

CONTENTS

ACKNOWLEDGMENTS

This book is not solely mine. It belongs to many people. So, to each and every writer who submitted a question, I thank you for your curiosity, your amazing imagination, and your dedication to getting it right. I have learned as much from researching and answering your questions as I hope you have from my answers.

To each and every reader, I hope this book answers some of your own questions, raises your level of understanding of medical and forensic issues, causes new questions to sprout within your own mind, and, most of all, stirs your creative juices.

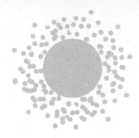

INTRODUCTION

My first Q&A book, *Murder and Mayhem: A Doctor Answers Medical and Forensic Questions for Mystery Writers,* appeared in 2003. Since then I have received many more fascinating and challenging questions from writers in all genres and from all parts of the world. With over a thousand questions to sift through, selecting which ones to place in this volume proved daunting. I must admit that I had fun rereading each question, editing the ones selected, and finally putting together a collection of questions that I believe are even more interesting than the ones that appeared in the first volume.

Sadly, hundreds of questions didn't make the cut, for no other reason than that space would not allow it. Each unused question was interesting, informative, and deserving, but had they been included, this book would easily have been twice its size.

This time I decided to do something a little different. I've attributed each question to its author, if he or she so chose. Some writers preferred to remain anonymous, and others I simply could not reach because their contact information was no longer valid.

You will see questions from professional, multipublished, award-winning authors alongside those submitted by writers who are hammering out their first work of fiction. What do these writers at different stages of their careers have in common? Each is a storyteller with a yarn to spin. Each possesses the same driving curiosity and the desire to get it right. Each settles in before a blank page or an empty computer screen with the same hopes: Can I craft a fun and believable story? Can I get what is in my head down on paper in a coherent manner? Can I make the reader turn the page?

Many of the questioners have books in publication as well as personal Web sites. Visit their sites and read their books. You'll be rewarded for your effort.

What This Book Is

As with *Murder and Mayhem,* my previous book, *Forensics and Fiction* is intended to inform and entertain not only writers, but also anyone who enjoys books, movies, or simply a good story. Reading through these questions and answers will offer some insight into how a writer works, by revealing what mental images he or she creates and what thought processes lead to constructing a story's plot. I am confident that readers will find many interesting, educational, humorous, and downright odd things inside.

In answering each question, I have attempted to give the writer enough background to add context to the particular medical or forensic issue at hand as well as to address the nuances of their particular scenario. The goal is to allow the writer to use this newly gained understanding to craft a more believable scene or story. I have attempted to make each question and answer stand alone while minimizing unnecessary repetition of information contained in other questions.

What This Book Is Not

In no way should the material contained in this publication be used for diagnosis or treatment of any medical disorder. Even the simplest question and answer would require decades of education and experience before it could be applied in a real-life situation.

Although I have endeavored to make the information accurate and scientifically correct, many subjects are too complex to explain in detail while addressing the nuances and controversies of modern medical knowledge. Such is the art of medicine. The answers are provided for use in the context of fiction writing and storytelling and should not be used for any other purpose.

This book is not to be used as a manual for any criminal activity or to bring harm to anyone.

Part I

Traumatic Injuries, Illnesses, Doctors, and Hospitals

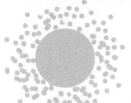

What Are the Symptoms and Signs of Bleeding to Death?

Q: What would be the symptoms and visible signs of being bled to death? The situation in my story is a man being bled to death by way of blood transfusion tubes.

Marion Arnott
Paisley, Scotland
Author of *Sleepwalkers*

A: Blood is a liquid filled with various cell types, one type being the red blood cells (RBCs). These contain hemoglobin, a molecule that carries oxygen (O_2) from the lungs to the tissues and removes carbon dioxide (CO_2) from the tissues and transports it to the lungs, where it is exhaled with each breath. Bleeding, depending upon how rapid it is, leads to two basic derangements. One is a drop in blood pressure (BP), resulting in shock, and the other is the development of anemia, which is a low level of RBCs in the blood. The former is due to a rapid drop in the volume of the blood (think bleeding air from a tire—as you do, the pressure within the tire falls) and the latter is due to a loss of the blood cells that carry oxygen.

In your scenario, if the blood is removed rapidly, the volume of blood in the victim's body falls, which causes a drop in BP, and results in shock and, if not treated appropriately and quickly, death. This is what happens when someone exsanguinates (bleeds to death) after an auto accident, a gunshot wound (GSW), or a rapidly bleeding ulcer. Depending upon the size of the person, the body contains from 8 to 12 pints of blood. The rapid loss of 3 or 4 pints would lead to shock in most people. So, if the blood were removed from your victim rapidly, his BP would fall and he would begin to show signs of shock.

These signs and symptoms include shortness of breath, weakness, dizziness, chills, thirst, and as it progresses, confusion, disorientation, sleepiness, coma, and death. This could happen over a few minutes or an hour or so, depending upon how rapidly the blood was removed.

If the bleeding is slow (your villain removing a little blood each day) the person will become progressively anemic. In anemia the RBC count is low, so the ability of the blood to transport O_2 to the body is reduced. Why? Less RBCs per ounce of blood means that each ounce of blood pumped by the heart carries less O_2. This means the tissues receive less O_2 and the symptoms of anemia reflect this reduction. They include shortness of breath (particularly with activity), fatigue, weakness, lethargy, headache, pallor (pale appearance), and chills. If your perpetrator bled your victim to death slowly, by removing blood little by little, these symptoms and signs would develop and progress as the anemia worsened. This could occur over many hours, days, or weeks.

How Long Might My Character Survive in a Cave with No Food or Water?

Q: A character in my story is trapped in a cool, dark cave with no food or water for several days. The gist of the story shows the rescuers trying to find him intercut with scenes of what he goes through emotionally and physically. He is in excellent physical shape, early twenties, but almost dies from the experience. How long would that take? Any gritty details?

Tammy Guest
Atlantis Project
Deydreem Productions

A: If your victim had a sufficient supply of good air, the major threats to his life would be dehydration and hypothermia (low body temperature). If he had enough warm clothing or materials to make clothing from, such as canvas or some other material, he would be able to avoid hypothermia for a longer period of time. If not, he would lose heat from his body fairly quickly. How quickly? That depends upon the actual temperature within the cave and whether the environment was damp or dry. Cold and wet would do him in more quickly.

The symptoms of hypothermia would be shivering, fatigue, weakness, and aching in his muscles and joints. As it progressed he would become lethargic, confused, and disoriented. He might even hallucinate. He would ultimately slip into a coma and die if not rescued. The presence of dehydration would magnify these symptoms.

Dehydration is sneaky and comes on at varying rates. If he is well hydrated at the beginning, has no significant medical problems, takes no dehydrating medications such as diuretics, does not consume alcohol, and doesn't overexert himself (sweating and heavy breathing take water from the body very quickly), it could take a couple of days before he showed signs of dehydration. It would then take several more days before he got into trouble, and a week or more before he was in danger of dying. It is highly variable, so this gives you great leeway in how you construct your story.

The symptoms of dehydration are similar to those of hypothermia. The general order of their appearance is: thirst, fatigue, weakness, shortness of breath, dizziness, disorientation, confusion, delusions, hallucinations, loss of consciousness, coma, and death. In a hot desert this sequence could play out in twelve hours, more or less. In your scenario it could take three to eight or so days, depending upon the above variables.

How Long Could a Child Survive in the Cold Waters Off the Coast of Maine?

Q: I'm writing about a twelve-year-old boy of average build who jumps out of a boat off the coast of Maine. The average water temperature in that area is approximately 55 degrees Fahrenheit. How many minutes could he live before dying of hypothermia?

A: Hypothermia onsets in the young and the old more quickly than it does in the average adult. Water temps in the mid 50s can definitely lead to hypothermia in a short period of time. The exact time is widely variable, depending upon such things as the victim's size, weight, percent of body fat, type of clothing, last meal, alcohol or drugs in the system, general health, and the movement of the water, to name a few. Large, obese, well-clothed people last longer. A recent large meal or alcohol intake will hasten heat loss, as will moving water. Think wind chill, only in the water. A cold stream or a choppy sea would remove body heat faster than would a calm cove.

You've no doubt heard of children drowning in frozen lakes and being pulled out forty-five minutes or more later and surviving without any problems. The reason is that the water is so cold (near freezing) that the metabolic processes in the body are slowed, and thus the body survives with no oxygen. This seems to occur only in children. But, your 55 degrees won't work in that fashion. That's just not low enough to "freeze" the body.

So, how long can your victim survive? The range is wide and could be as little as five minutes and as long as an hour. Average would be fifteen to thirty minutes in most circumstances.

What Duration of Exposure to High Environmental Temperatures Would Prove Lethal for a Pregnant Woman?

Q: In my story, a pregnant lady in her mid thirties, roughly five weeks prior to her due date, is left bound and gagged in a non-air-conditioned dump somewhere just outside of Las Vegas. Assuming she and her unborn baby are in perfect health and temperatures in Vegas are around 90 degrees Fahrenheit, how long could this woman go before she's in danger of either dying or losing her baby? What might be the logical sequence of her deterioration over a ten-hour time span under these conditions?

> Gar Anthony Haywood (writing as Ray Shannon)
> Los Angeles, California
> Shamus- and Anthony-award-winning author of *Man Eater* and *Firecracker*
> www.garanthonyhaywood.com

A: Exposure to this level of temperature, particularly in a very dry climate such as Las Vegas, would rapidly lead to dehydration, and then heat prostration and heatstroke. Collectively these three derangements are termed "heat injuries." When the body is exposed to extremes of temperature, breathing and sweating increase in an attempt to lower the body's core temperature. This leads to dehydration. As water loss from the body progresses, the body's core temperature begins to rise and sweating increases. The blood pressure (BP) then begins to drop, the heart rate increases, and the body temperature can reach as high as 104 or 105 degrees. This is termed heat prostration. Further along in this process the severe dehydration and high body temperature causes damage to the brain, particularly the area we call the hypothalamus, which controls body temperature regulation. When this happens sweating ceases and the core temperature may soar to 106–108 or higher. This is called heatstroke, and is a true medical emergency. If the body temperature is not quickly lowered and the victim rehydrated, the brain will be permanently damaged and death will follow.

The 90-degree heat, low humidity, and your unfortunate young lady's inability to reach a water source would lead to rapid dehydration. She would experience thirst, shortness of breath, fatigue, headache, and dizziness. As she developed heat prostration, each of these symptoms would be magnified, and she would experience confusion, disorientation, delusions, and visual or auditory hallucinations. That is, she would see and hear bizarre things. As she slipped into heatstroke, coma, seizures, and shock would follow, culminating in her death.

All these changes would be more serious and would come on more rapidly in a pregnant woman, since her cardiovascular system would already be under stress from the pregnancy. By ten hours she would be severely dehydrated, and could even enter heat prostration or heatstroke, though the latter two would probably take eighteen to thirty-six hours to develop. This varies widely from person to person, so if after ten hours she were only dehydrated, that would be realistic. Or, if she developed one of the more severe forms of heat injury, or even if she died, this would also be possible and believable. You can have it any way you need for your story.

When rescued, her treatment would be directed toward lowering the core temperature as quickly as possible. Moving her to a shaded, well-ventilated area and pouring water over her while fanning her with a towel could be life saving. If able to swallow, she would be given water to drink. She would then be transported to the hospital, where IV fluids and further cooling measures, such as a cooling blanket (a synthetic drape through which cold water is circulated) or an ice bath, would be instituted.

She and her baby could survive unscathed, or one or both of them could suffer severe brain damage, or one or both of them could die. Any of these scenarios is possible.

How Would a Heart Attack Be Treated During a Commercial Plane Flight?

Q: One of my characters is a sixty-five-year-old married man who has angina, for which he takes nitroglycerin. I want to give him a nonfatal heart attack during a commercial plane flight from Tampa to New York City. He's treated on an emergency basis by the flight attendants or a physician passenger. When he gets to New York City he's taken to a hospital and is told he needs a quadruple bypass. He refuses to get the bypass right away (for story reasons), and then has another attack, is taken back to the hospital, and is near death for a while.

Finally he agrees to have the surgery. Will this sequence of events work? What actually happens on the plane and at the hospital?

M. Diane Vogt

Tampa, Florida

www.mdianevogt.com

A: The scenario you lay out is not uncommon. Men refuse the proper medical care all the time. They are often pigheaded when it comes to health. It's that Superman thing.

On the plane he would develop chest pain, shortness of breath, nausea, and diaphoresis (become sweaty). The flight attendants would ask if any M.D. was on the flight, and if so he would help with the man's care. They would give him oxygen, lay him down in the rear of the plane, and divert the flight to the nearest major airport. So have this happen near New York if that's where you want the story to occur. Otherwise he might end up in Atlanta, Washington D.C., or wherever the nearest major city is.

Airlines have emergency kits and, using one, the M.D. could start an intravenous line (IV) and attach the onboard cardiac monitor. If the victim suffered a cardiac arrest, the doctor would immediately begin CPR, and hopefully the plane would be equipped with an AED (automatic external defibrillator). If so, this would be attached to the victim, using sticky disklike electrodes that would be placed on his chest. The AED has a computer that reads the cardiac rhythm. If he developed the deadly rhythms called "ventricular tachycardia" (V-Tach or VT) or "ventricular fibrillation" (V-Fib or VF), the AED would deliver an electric shock to hopefully snap the heart back into a normal rhythm.

Once in the hospital he would be taken to the ICU where an electrocardiogram (EKG) and blood work would show that he had had a heart attack (myocardial infarction, or MI). He would go to the catheterization lab for a coronary angiogram, which would reveal multivessel coronary artery disease (CAD), and surgery would be recommended. After he refused and had another MI, he would be in an even more precarious situation, and might then agree to the surgery. Seen it a thousand times.

Can an Automobile Accident Victim Suffer Amnesia for Ten Days and Then Suddenly Recover Her Memory?

Q: My victim and her friend are in a car accident in which the friend, who is driving, dies instantly, and the victim survives but is in a coma for a brief period. When she awakens, she has no memory of the accident, but ten days later her memory returns. She can then tell the police that her friend was trying to use her brakes, which failed, rather than simply running a red light. Is this realistic? Also, what type of injury would cause this, and what testing and treatment would she undergo when she arrived at the hospital? Would there be any long-term effects of her injuries?

A: Yes, all of this will work for your story. Comas and amnesia are funny things, and virtually anything can happen.

Her injury would most likely be blunt trauma to the head from the dashboard or the windshield. She could or could not suffer a skull fracture, but that's not necessary for her to be in a coma for a couple of days or to develop the amnesia you need for your story.

A comatose person may remain so for days or months or years and then wake up gradually, in fits and spurts, or suddenly. After awakening she would likely be somewhat confused and disoriented for a period of time. This could be minutes, hours, days, or weeks, after which she could return completely to normal or could be left with various mental deficits such as confusion and disorientation. She could also have a wide range of personality changes. She could be withdrawn, talkative and outgoing, paranoid, angry and combative, or any combination of these. Or she could simply wake up and be normal in every respect. All is possible.

She would have no memory for the time she was comatose and may or may not remember what came before. This is called retrograde amnesia. This retrograde loss of memory could go back any period of time before the accident—a few minutes, a few hours, days, months, years, or forever. And her memory of previous events could be partial, spotty, or complete. It may return slowly over days, weeks, or months, or may return quickly. Again, all is possible.

The bottom line is that coma and amnesia are both poorly understood and come in thousands of flavors. This is good for you, since you can craft your story any way you wish and it will work.

When she got to the hospital she would go through a battery of tests designed to find out if she had any serious brain injury. These could include skull X-rays, CT scans, MRIs, and EEGs (an EEG is an electroencephalogram—a measure of brain wave activity). When the tests all came back normal, the diagnosis would be a cerebral contusion (basically a brain bruise). She would be given steroids, such as Decadron or Solu-Medrol, to lessen any brain swelling. Other than that, time would be the only treatment.

Once she woke up the M.D. would perform complete neurological and mental status exams to assess brain function. This is complex, and I doubt you really need it for your story. If all went well, she might go home a few days after awakening, and she might not require any long-term treatment. Or she could need a period of physical therapy and psychiatric counseling. The most likely long-term symptom she would have is a few weeks of headaches.

Can a Head Injury Cause the Loss of Memory for Things That Happened Before the Injury?

Q: I am working on a story where the main character was raped and had a child as a result of the rape. A couple of years later she's in an accident and loses her memory after hitting her head. She's unconscious for a short time, and when she wakes up, she doesn't know her child, and her memory goes back only two years. Is it plausible that she would wake and not remember the rape and her child? I have a great idea worked out, but this needs to be plausible or the idea won't work. Any thoughts?

Nikki Leigh
Author of *Stormy View*
www.nikkileigh.com

A: Your scenario is very plausible. Our memories are fragile and can be affected by many things, including trauma, both physical and psychological.

Amnesia, or the loss of memory, can be only for the time period that the victim is unconscious or it can be anterograde or retrograde. What you are describing is retrograde amnesia. This is a loss of memory of things that happened before the injury. Anterograde amnesia is trickier and not common. Here the injury does something to the brain that makes the victim unable to form new memories. The person could remember things that happened before the injury but could not form any new memories and would quickly forget what happened five minutes ago. This type of amnesia is central to the plot of the movie *Memento*. A very clever story.

Memory is funny, and can do almost anything. Which is good news for your story, in that anything can happen so you can have it any way you want it. The retrograde amnesia you need for your character could be complete or partial. That is, she could remember some things and not others, or she could remember nothing at all. It could be for any past time period and could be brief, or of a long duration, or permanent. It could return suddenly, slowly, in bits and pieces, or not at all. The return of her memory could be triggered by something she sees, hears, smells, touches, or tastes. A word in a conversation, an image on TV, an object she picks up, a song on the radio, or the odor of something noxious or of an old favorite food could each be the trigger. Anything is possible.

How Long Could a Man Survive in the Desert After Major Injuries from an Automobile Accident?

Q: Here's my scenario: A man loses control of his SUV and drives off a cliff on a remote dirt road outside of Kingman, Arizona. Nobody notices the accident. He breaks his pelvis, maybe his legs, maybe a couple of ribs. Due to his injuries he is unable to climb back up the hill to the road. He survives on water from his windshield wiper reservoir, and eats bugs and lizards and whatever else he can find. He uses the wreckage for shelter in the sweltering heat and isn't found for five or six days.

What condition would he be in? Dehydrated? Badly sunburned? Unconscious? What would he look like? Once the guy is back in the hospital in Kingman, what treatment would they give him?

Lee Goldberg

Los Angeles, California

Author of the Diagnosis Murder and Monk series

www.leegoldberg.com

A: Yes, he would be severely dehydrated. More so if the temperature was high, as it is in summer there, and less so if in winter. In fact, in winter he could die from hypothermia.

If he broke his pelvis and/or a leg or two there would be some internal bleeding, which would only add to his problem. If he then had only a little water and some berries and bugs he would become severely dehydrated, and would likely slip into shock and could die. But you want him to survive, so a pelvic fracture would work well. Or a fracture to his lower leg. The bones there are the tibia (big one) and the fibula (little one). I would not have him fracture his femur (upper leg bone), since this is often associated with a great deal of internal bleeding into the leg, and his survival under the conditions you describe would be much less likely. A pelvic fracture might prevent him from climbing or crawling back up to the road and would limit his mobility greatly.

Dehydration is the loss of body water. The rate at which we lose water depends upon several factors, such as the ambient temperature (the higher it is, the faster the loss from sweating), activity (water is lost through the lungs with each breath, and exercise increases breathing), medications or drugs (alcohol and diuretics both cause water loss through the kidneys), and other factors. The symptoms of dehydration are thirst, fatigue, dry mouth, nausea, sleepiness, confusion, disorientation, and finally shock (low blood pressure), a rise in body temperature, and then death, more or less in that order of appearance. He may also hallucinate or see mirages, which are due to a bending of light rays. The heat rising from a desert bends light rays due to changes in the density of the air. The result is that you see blue sky below the horizon, and it looks like a body of water. Often a person who is dehydrated and confused will rush (with your character, crawl) blindly toward it, but can never reach it because it doesn't exist, and because the optical illusion keeps moving away.

The rapidity with which dehydration occurs will dictate how quickly these symptoms appear and how severe they are. Organ damage is primarily to the kidneys, which can be severely and irreversibly damaged with severe or prolonged dehydration.

In your scenario the dehydration would come on slowly, over a day or two, and would not become severe for as much as three or four days. Of course, if he lost considerable blood from his injuries, this process would occur much more quickly. Also, at higher altitudes dehydration comes on more rapidly because the air at high altitudes tends to be drier. This means that more water is lost through the lungs than is lost in damper air at sea level. Kingman is fairly high and dry. His movements as he crawled around and searched for food would also dehydrate him more quickly.

Since your victim is young and healthy, and I assume is not taking any diuretics and has not consumed any alcohol before the beginning of his ordeal, two days would be a good average time frame for him to get into trouble but survive without major problems. You could stretch this to three or four days if necessary, but no longer. Not in the sweltering heat you described. Otherwise he could develop heat prostration or heatstroke, and die.

When found he could be awake and alert, confused and disoriented, or in a coma. All of these are possible. The rescuers would wrap him in a blanket if he were cold, or douse him with water and fan him if he were suffering heat prostration or heatstroke. They would give him sips of water, stabilize any leg fractures with splints, and call for help. Once in the hospital he would get IV fluids and X-rays. Blood work would be done to determine how much blood he had lost and to check for kidney problems from the dehydration. He could require a blood transfusion, and his leg or pelvis could need surgical repair. This would depend upon the type and extent of the fracture. Or he could need neither.

Yes, he could be sunburned unless he remained in his shelter during the day and searched for food at dawn and dusk.

Where Can My Character Be Shot and Survive but Be Partially Disabled?

Q: In my story I need a female cop in her early thirties to get shot four times at close range with a .22 caliber handgun, and live to tell about it. Her injuries must be sufficient to end her police career, but not to take her life. She might come out of the shooting with a slight physical impairment (limp, partial use of one arm/hand, etc.), but without any loss of her mental capacities. Could you please give me a hypothetical regarding:
  • Where her four bullet wounds could be sustained, and the damage done?
  • What kind of physical therapy she might have to undergo afterward?
  • How long it might take her to get back on her feet again?

Gar Anthony Haywood (writing as Ray Shannon)
Los Angeles, California

Shamus- and Anthony-award-winning author of
Man Eater and *Firecracker*
www.garanthonyhaywood.com

A: A .22 caliber pistol is among the least destructive handguns. The bullet is small and relatively slow. Still, it can cause significant injury, and even death.

Your victim could be shot almost anywhere and survive. A shot to the head, chest, abdomen, or anywhere else does not necessarily lead to death. The bullet can simply lodge beneath the skin or strike a bone or rib or skull and be deflected away from vital organs. So three of the four bullets could be flesh wounds, and the fourth could do the damage.

She could be shot in the chest near the shoulder, and the one bullet that caused major harm could damage her brachial plexus. This is the bundle of blood vessels and nerves that leaves the chest and enters the arm through the axilla (armpit). The nerves come from the spinal cord through the axilla and supply all areas of the arm and hand. They carry sensory fibers (feeling/sensations) and motor fibers (stimulate muscle movements). The subclavian artery branches off the aorta, passes through the axilla, and supplies blood to the arm. Damage to either the nerves or the artery could require surgery to remove the bullet and repair the damaged blood vessels or nerves. This type of injury could easily leave her with some degree of disability such as weakness, numbness, and perhaps long-term pain in the arm on that side.

She would receive physical therapy (PT) and occupational therapy (OT) in the form of strength and coordination training. PT would consist of resistance exercises and stretching, and range-of-motion exercises to improve the strength and mobility of the arm and hand. OT would consist of finger and hand activities (finger tapping, dexterity exercises, even playing the piano) to regain or at least improve the function of her hand and fingers. OT is designed so that the person can regain what we call "fine motor skills." These are things like writing, picking up small objects, turning doorknobs, brushing hair, working with her hands and fingers, and all other daily activities of life.

This disability would likely end her career—at least as a patrol officer—and her PT and OT could take months.

She would be back on her feet a few days after surgery, but her return to full function could take months. Or she may never regain full use of her arm and hand, and might be retired from the force, or at least given a desk job.

What Happens When Someone Is Shot in the Heart with an Arrow?

Q: If a character shoots an arrow into someone's chest, what would the area around the wound look like (amount of blood, spatter, etc.)? Presuming the arrow hit the heart, how long would it take that person to die? Would the heart stop, or would it keep pumping, with the victim then bleeding out?

Twist Phelan

Author of the Pinnacle Peak mystery series

www.twistphelan.com

A: An arrow to the heart may or may not be lethal. If it is lethal, it will kill in one of several ways. The penetration of the heart muscle by the arrow could set off a lethal abnormal cardiac rhythm, usually ventricular fibrillation (VF) or ventricular tachycardia (VT). In this case the victim would suddenly collapse and die. There would be some bleeding, but not a great deal. When the heart goes into VF or VT, or when it stops, it no longer pumps blood and the wound ceases to bleed.

The arrow could damage the heart's muscle or valves in such a way that it is no longer effective as a pump. The blood pressure (BP) would fall; the victim would slip into shock and die. Here the death would take a few minutes, and there would be some bleeding, but still not likely a great deal. At least, not externally.

The arrow could enter the heart muscle but do little real damage. Here the bleeding from the puncture could collect in the pericardium (the sac around the heart) and produce what is called "tamponade." The pericardium is not compliant (stretchy or expandable), so as blood accumulates within it the pressure within the pericardium will rise. Think of it as an overinflated tire. This increased pressure will squeeze the heart to the point that it can no longer pump blood. Again, the BP would gradually fall, and the victim would slip into shock and die. This could take a couple of minutes to an hour, or anywhere in between.

Or the arrow could penetrate the heart and there could be little bleeding, either internally or externally. The arrow would serve as the finger in the dike, so to speak. The victim could walk into the ER with an arrow in his heart. It would gently waggle with each heartbeat. I've seen this with an ice pick, but not with an arrow.

Finally, the arrow could penetrate the heart but not set off a deadly arrhythmia or severely damage the heart, and either fall out or be pulled out. Here there would be more external bleeding than if the arrow remained in place, since nothing would prevent the heart from pumping blood through the hole where the arrow had been. This would be the bloodiest scenario. The blood would gush through the hole with each heartbeat, diminishing in volume minute by minute, until the victim bled out or the heart stopped. This would take only a very few minutes, since the victim would fairly quickly slip into shock and die.

So the arrow can kill quickly with little bleeding, more slowly with some bleeding (still not a great deal), slowly with more bleeding if the arrow fell out, or it could remain in place and not kill at all. Any of these and many other scenarios are possible.

How Is a Gunshot to the Hand Treated?

Q: My protagonist, a police investigator, has two fingers of her right hand, the index and middle fingers, shot off. How would she be bandaged? Would she be in a sling and need to keep the hand elevated? How long before she could return to work? Would she still "feel" the two missing fingers?

Gay Toltl Kinman
Alhambra, California
Author of *Castle Reiner* and *Super Sleuth: Five Alison Leigh Powers Mysteries*
gaykinman.com

A: The hand would be cleaned and dressed with antibiotic ointments, and then would be formed into a fist around a wad of sterile gauze. The entire hand would then be wrapped. It would look like a boxing glove. This claw-shaped positioning of the hand is termed the "position of function," and it allows for faster and better healing. It would be elevated to reduce swelling, and when she was up and about it would be placed in a sling. It would be treated in this fashion for about a week, and then the wound would be covered with a smaller bandage—no balling of the fist—for another week or so. The entire healing process would take four to six weeks. She could return to desk work in a week or two, and to full duty, limited only by her now handicapped condition, after about two months or so.

The sensation that her fingers are still present is called "phantom sensation" and, if painful, "phantom pain." She could feel either or both, but more likely neither. Phantom sensations do happen but are not common.

What Are the Symptoms of a Ruptured Brain Aneurysm?

Q: In the early part of my novel a character dies from a brain aneurysm. Her death becomes a catalyst for my main character. I know these are often associated with severe headaches, but how long would her headache last before she died? Would she die suddenly? Would she be conscious till the end?

Kimberly Burton Allen
Southampton, New York
Author of *A Butler's Life: Scenes from the Other Side of the Silver Salver*

A: An aneurysm is a swelling of an artery, and can occur anywhere in the body. The brain is a common place for them to occur. These are typically round or fusiform (football-shaped), but some brain aneurysms are saclike swellings, which look like berries hanging from a plant stem. These are called, as you would likely guess, "berry aneurysms." Regardless of the shape, this swelling thins the wall of the artery, and it may leak or rupture.

If an aneurysm leaks, the resulting bleeding is slow, and the symptoms are typically a mild to severe headache, and possibly nausea, vomiting, photophobia (intolerance to light), numbness and weakness of a limb or the face, sleepiness, confusion, disorientation. The accumulation of blood within or around the brain causes a marked increase in pressure within the skull, since it does not expand. This will compress the respiratory (breathing) area of the brain, and may cause a cessation of breathing, and death. Or not. The bleeding may stop, and the person may recover without any treatment or long-term problems.

If an aneurysm ruptures it produces an even more dangerous situation. Here the bleeding is more sudden and extensive, and the pressure within the skull rises rapidly. Headache is usually sudden and severe, and coma, cessation of breathing, and death may occur very quickly.

Or anywhere in between these two extremes.

In your scenario the victim could suffer one of several common sequences of events. The bleeding could be sudden and brisk, and she would develop a sudden headache, perhaps localized in one temple or behind one eye, collapse, maybe suffer a seizure (or not), and die. Sudden and dramatic. Or she could develop a headache that waxed and waned, or that progressed slowly over hours or days. She could become nauseated and develop any of the above symptoms. She might take over-the-counter headache meds with little relief. If she used aspirin, which is a blood thinner, she could make the bleeding more severe, the headache more severe, and death more likely. She might lie down to take a nap and never wake up. Or after several days or hours of headaches she could suddenly collapse and die.

The bottom line is that this medical problem has many faces, which means you have great leeway in how you create your scene.

What Happens During a Suicide by Hanging?

Q: In my work in progress a twelve-year-old girl attempts suicide by hanging. She is found before she dies. What are the physiological phases between kicking the ladder out, losing consciousness, and death? Is it possible for her to be discovered and saved or revived (undamaged), and how quickly must this occur?

A: In hangings death results from asphyxia, which is the reduction of oxygen to the brain. This results from the compression of the airways and the carotid arteries by the noose, which is pulled tight by the body weight. The carotid arteries lie on either side of the neck and carry blood to the brain. Though the airway can be obstructed and breathing interrupted, the real cause of loss of consciousness and death in most hangings is compression of the arteries, which blocks blood flow to the brain. Except for judicial (legally directed) hangings, fractures of the cervical vertebrae (spinal bones of the neck) are uncommon.

In suicidal hangings the victim typically uses whatever is handy for a noose. Ropes, belts, bedsheets, clothing, and electrical cords are common. Occasionally the victim will bind her own hands to prevent a change of heart. This is an important fact, since the finding of bound hands would seem to indicate that the hanging was a homicide, or at least that the victim had recruited some help in her suicide. This is simply not the case. Of course, the binding must be such that the victim could have done it herself. Otherwise, homicide is a possibility. If the victim does not tie her own hands, she may attempt to undo the noose, and there may be scratches and gouges of the flesh near the noose.

Since the asphyxia is due to compression of the arteries and not the prevention of breathing, loss of consciousness occurs very quickly, usually in a minute or less, and maybe in as little as twenty seconds. The brain needs a continuous supply of blood, and when this is interrupted, consciousness is lost quickly. Death may take from one to five or six minutes, and children seem to "tolerate" hanging for a longer time period than adults.

If your victim were found within a couple of minutes, she would be unconscious but could wake up fairly quickly once the noose was removed. She would probably have the typical V-shaped bruises of hanging on her neck. She would be taken to the hospital ER, where she would be evaluated with X-rays of her neck, and perhaps a neurologist would be called in to determine if she had suffered any brain damage. She could return completely to normal, or be left with brain damage, or even remain in a coma for hours, days, weeks, months, years, or forever. It all depends upon how long the brain was deprived of blood and the victim's tolerance for such deprivation. This varies greatly from person to person.

A psychiatrist would definitely be involved following any suicide attempt, and the victim would be kept in the hospital until he determined that it was safe for her to go home. The doctor has the legal right and the ethical responsibility to keep her under observation regardless of what the victim and her parents want. That is, the parents could demand that she be released to them, but legally the hospital can keep her until it is determined that she is no longer a threat to herself. Also, the police would be involved since hanging can be part of or as a result of child abuse. Sadly, sometimes children see this as the only way out of an abusive situation.

How Does the So-Called Flesh-Eating Bacteria Harm Humans?

Q: For a short story I need to ask a few questions about the so-called flesh-eating bacteria. I understand that bacteria are all around us, and that they like to invade open wounds. What causes this strain of bacteria to attack some people but not others? Can flesh-eating bacteria actually be seen on a victim? That is, can they grow to such numbers that they become visible to the naked eye

(like molds)? Can they also attack orifices in addition to
wounds?

Lyn Tucker
Carlsbad, California

A: There are several species of bacteria that can become flesh eating. The term simply means that the bacteria are aggressive and
cause widespread tissue destruction as they grow. The one that has
captured the public's attention in recent years is a strain of *Strepto-
coccus*. This strain typically invades open wounds, multiplies rapidly,
and produces enzymes that cause destruction of tissues. Why would
it do this? Simply put, the bacteria use the tissues for nutrition, thus
they are flesh eating. The enzymes liquefy the tissues, allowing the
bacteria to more easily "digest" the nutrients in the flesh, which
enables the bacteria to thrive and multiply. It's not really different
from what occurs in our own gastrointestinal tract when we take in
food. Enzymes within our digestive system break down carbohy-
drates, fats, and proteins into usable units, which are then absorbed
into the bloodstream and carried to all the body's cells. The flesh-
eating bacteria are simply doing the same thing.

The body has several layers of defense against microorganisms.
The skin acts as a barrier, the various types of white blood cells
(WBCs) act as warriors and scavengers, and the immune system
possesses very elegant mechanisms for attacking and weakening
unwanted invaders, making them easy prey for the scavenging
WBCs. Any breach or compromise in these layers of defense opens
the door to invasion and infection. A break in the skin barrier
allows entry. Defective white blood cells, as is seen in many types
of leukemia and lymphoma, weaken the defensive lines. Any compromise in the immune system, as is seen in HIV/AIDS and people
who are on immunosuppressive therapy after organ transplant, or
in the presence of diseases such as diabetes, increases the chance of
infection. For these reasons one person may get the flu or pneumonia or a flesh-eating bacterial infection while the next person
will not. A person with a normal immune system and white blood
cells will not likely become infected around any of his bodily orifices unless some breach in the skin barrier is present. In compro-

mised persons infections of the mouth and urinary tract are all too common. And can be deadly.

Bacteria are microscopic and cannot be seen with the naked eye. The infection will produce reddening and swelling of the infected flesh, and pus (basically dead WBCs and bacteria), which are visible.

Can My Character Fake Being Blind?

Q: I have a plot question regarding blindness. A female character is the ringleader of a criminal gang, and is supposedly blind. In reality, she is not. She is married to an honest man who knows nothing about her fake blindness or her illegal activities. Is there a way to fake blindness convincingly? Are there any drops that do not harm the eye but keep the pupils from reacting to light, or are there any medical conditions that can result in partial to full blindness but depend on the honest responses of the person afflicted to determine the true range of vision?

A: Blindness has little to do with pupillary reactions. Let me explain.

Vision depends on light entering the eye through the pupil and striking the retina in the back of the eyeball. This causes a chemical reaction, which in turn sends an electrical impulse through the optic nerve to the brain, where it is processed to create a "picture." A failure at any step in this chain of events can result in altered vision or complete blindness.

The pupils are involved in vision only in that they regulate the amount of light that comes in—dilated (enlarged) in dim lighting, and constricted (small) in bright lighting—and have little relation to whether the person sees or not. Many blind persons retain normal pupillary reactivity, so this is not a test for blindness.

There are many forms of true blindness. Some involve the eye itself, others the optic nerve, and still others are what we term "cortical blindness." The cortex is the outer covering of the brain, and different areas of it are involved in different neurological activities. The part that deals with vision is the occipital cortex, which is the very back part of the brain. Strokes or injuries to this area can cause blindness, which may be partial or complete, temporary or permanent.

There is also a psychiatric condition known as "hysterical blindness." This often follows a severe psychological trauma, and the victim will not be able to see. Not for any physical reason but due to a psychological block.

If your faker is good, it may be very difficult or impossible to determine if she is blind or not. However, if someone were to toss something at her or pretend to strike her in the face, and if she reacted, her fakery would be exposed. A truly blind person would not see anything and would not react. She could still pull it off, but only if no one actually challenged her in this fashion.

How can you get around this? Give her partial blindness. There are several possibilities, but one that I would suggest: bilateral retinal detachments. This is where the retina begins to separate from the eyeball, and if untreated can lead to permanent blindness or visual impairment. The bilateral form affects both eyes. This can happen in diabetes, with high blood pressure, after trauma, and sometimes for no known reason.

She could tell people that she has this problem and is nearly blind, but not completely. She could say she is legally blind, which means that her vision is so impaired that she can't read, watch TV, or drive a car. She might say that she can see light, colors, vague shapes, and shadows but little else. In this case, if someone challenged her as described above, her natural reaction could be explained. She would see "something" moving toward her.

She could wear dark glasses, use a cane, and might need help with walking, be driven around, have papers read to her, etc. She could say that she was going to have laser surgery to try to correct it, but it couldn't be done for a while. Maybe not until some bleeding and swelling resolved, for example. Or she could say that her doctor told her she was not a candidate for such a procedure and that her problem was permanent.

She could easily pull off this scam because it is not a rare occurrence, and it would garner a great deal of sympathy, even from her enemies.

How and for What Purpose Was the Ancient Practice of Bloodletting Performed?

Q: For my story I'm looking for some particularly barbaric or stupid medical practice from the 1800s that I can use as an example of backward, outdated medicine that would defy common sense now. I was considering something like the ancient practice of bleeding people to make them healthy. How and why was this done?

Lee Goldberg
Los Angeles, California
Author of the Diagnosis Murder and Monk series
www.leegoldberg.com

A: Yes, bloodletting would do it. It was widely used from the time of Galen (the first century B.C.) until the late nineteenth century, and even into the twentieth. A surgeon would use a blade or lancet to open a vein, and the blood would be collected. As much as two or three pints were sometimes removed at one time, though usually less was taken. But the procedure might have been repeated over several days, so three or more pints would ultimately be taken. It is a testament to the toughness of humans that more didn't die of shock. It was used for fevers, dropsy (edema or swelling), consumption (TB), and almost every other disease known.

Dropsy was the term used until the mid-twentieth century for edema or swelling of the ankles, legs, and in severe cases the entire body. Usually it was due to heat and/or kidney failure. We now call this congestive heart failure or renal (kidney) failure. In this situation the body is overloaded with salt and water, the lungs fill with water, and the victim dies of asphyxia, basically drowning from wet lungs. Now we use diuretics to remove water via the kidneys, and in the case of severe kidney failure, dialysis. In the case of dropsy, bloodletting was likely life saving. So even though it was used without any understanding of physiology, sometimes the ancients got lucky. And bloodletting is not as outdated as most people believe.

When I was in medical school we used phlebotomy (taking blood from a vein) in cases of severe, acute heart failure and pulmonary edema (lungs full of water) as a life-saving measure while waiting for the diuretics to work. These drugs may require an hour or so to take full effect, and the patient could die in the interim. Phlebotomy is the removal of blood a pint at a time as needed to relieve the pulmonary edema. This is basically bloodletting. Since we have more powerful diuretics today, this is rarely used anymore.

If a doctor in your story used it for anything other than heart or renal failure, it would indeed be barbaric and stupid. And even if he used it for heart or renal failure in place of more standard treatments, it would raise an eyebrow or two.

How Long Might My Comatose Character Survive?

Q: I am writing a novel in which the protagonist's thirty-five-year-old wife is in a coma after a head injury sustained in a hit-and-run car accident. She never regains consciousness, and ultimately dies. I want her to be in a vegetative state that does not necessitate life-support machinery. What medical complications might she die from, and how long might she be expected to live?

> Trisha Rainsford
> Limerick, Ireland
> Author of *The Knack of Life* and coauthor of
> *Hot Property*, a Sarah O'Brien novel

A: Many people in a permanent vegetative state require no life support, only feeding and general care. They can survive for decades with proper care. The major medical problems associated with this situation are:

Bedsores: These are actually pressure sores that result when a body lies unmoving for extended periods. These sores can be deep, even down to the bones, and can become infected. If they do they can be very difficult to treat, and can lead to septicemia (infection in the bloodstream), which can cause death.

Pneumonia: This is an infection in the lungs that is common in coma victims. A person in a coma doesn't breathe as deeply as one who is awake and active; the lungs can collapse slightly, and an infection can easily occur. These infections can be difficult to treat, and deadly. Also, pneumonias often occur after aspiration of liquid foods, which are typically given to comatose individuals by way of a feeding tube. People in comas are not able to eat, so a tube for feeding is passed through the nose and into the stomach, and left there. The presence of such a feeding tube increases the probability that acids and food materials from the stomach can rise into the esophagus (swallowing tube) and enter the lungs. The acids can then actually burn the lungs and the bronchial (breathing) tubes, and allow infections with some pretty nasty bugs to occur. This type of pneumonia is called aspiration pneumonia, and is very treacherous. One way to lessen this is with a gastrostomy tube. Here the plastic feeding tube is actually passed into the stomach through the abdominal wall rather than down the throat. This requires only a minor incision, and can stay for years. Since the tube does not pass through the throat, the incidence of aspiration is less.

Urinary tract infections: Many people in this circumstance will have a Foley catheter passed into the bladder to prevent them from soiling themselves. This tube can allow bacteria to enter the bladder, and then the kidneys. Again, these can seed the bloodstream and cause deadly septicemia.

Pulmonary embolus: This is a common and deadly complication. Here a blood clot forms in the veins of the legs or the pelvis, breaks off, and travels through the right side of the heart and into the lungs. This can lead to death in minutes. People who are immobile for any reason, such as someone in a coma or after an operation or a stroke, are very prone to this development.

So your character could live for decades, years, months, weeks, or days, and could die from an infection or a pulmonary embolism at any time. This means that you have a wide range to work with, and any of these times would be accurate and believable.

Does Salt Water Make a Good Antibacterial Agent?

Q: In my story a character suffers a knife wound, a slice across the forearm, while far from civilization. Another character treats it with seawater, and later, after they reach their campsite, with boiled water to which she has added salt, saying that this will keep the wound from getting infected. Is this true, or will my character sound ignorant?

A: No, your character is actually quite smart. Though salt water is not the best antibacterial, it is better than nothing. Mainly it cleans dirt and debris from the wound, which is very important in preventing infection. Also, it has some antibacterial qualities. The seawater would serve to clean the wound, and upon returning to camp, the boiled water with a higher concentration of salt could actually kill bacteria. Bacteria don't survive in very salty conditions. She could put two or three tablespoons of salt in a cup of water and irrigate the wound with it, then apply the cleanest bandage available. A piece of white cotton, boiled in water and then allowed to air dry, would be best.

Will a Child from an Incestuous Pregnancy Likely Have a Birth Defect?

Q: A character in my short story is pregnant (too far along for a legal abortion) and she discovers that the father of her child is actually her maternal grandfather. Will the baby likely be born with serious defects as a result of the incest?

> Susanne Shaphren
>
> Phoenix, Arizona
>
> Author of "Arrangements," in *Mystery Writers of America Presents Show Business Is Murder*, and "The Best of Friends," in *Sex, Lies, & Private Eyes*

A: Incest leads to genetic problems most frequently via recessive genes. All of our genes are paired, and in each pair one gene is typically dominant and the other recessive. The dominant one is the one that is expressed. For example, if you have two brown-eye genes you will have brown eyes, and if you have two blue-eye genes you will have blue eyes. But if you have one gene for brown eyes and one for blue eyes, you will likely have brown eyes. The blue-eye gene is recessive and the brown-eye gene is dominant. It isn't exactly this simple, but this should illustrate the point.

The same is true for certain diseases that are due to recessive genes. If you have a dominant gene and a recessive gene you will either not have the disease or you will have a milder form of it. But if you have two of the recessive genes the disease will appear, since there is no dominant gene to block or attenuate its expression. For example, the gene for normal hemoglobin (the oxygen-carrying molecule within our red blood cells, or RBCs) is usually designated as A. The gene for sickle cell anemia, a disease that predominantly affects those of African descent, is recessive to the A gene and is designated as S. Most people have a pair of genes that are normal, or AA. Those with what is called "sickle cell trait," the mild form of the disease, have one of each, and are designated AS. To have full-blown sickle cell anemia (SCA) the person would have to have two S genes, or be SS. Since one gene comes from each parent, a person with SCA must receive one of the S genes from each parent. This means that each parent must be either SS or AS. They must have an S gene to donate to the offspring.

That's sort of basic genetics. But as you can see, if a family has the S gene in its bloodline it is more likely to produce an SS child from a union between two family members than it would be if one parent came from the S gene–containing family and the other came from a bloodline that had no S genes in its pedigree.

This is true for all types of genetic disorders. Still, even with all this it is not common for a single episode of incest to produce a severely abnormal child. If the inbreeding continues over several generations, the recessive genes within that family become more plentiful within the group, and the incidents of significant genetic abnormalities increase accordingly.

So, for your story it is unlikely that the child would be harmed, but the character wouldn't know that. And even if the odds were 1 in 1,000, she would obsess about the 1 and not the 999. Her concerns would be real to her, and she would feel fear, anxiety, shame, regret, and all the other emotions that typically are associated with an incestuous relationship. And she would feel more so as her delivery date approached for fear that her secret would be discovered when she delivered a three-headed baby. In other words, her fear of the possibility is much more important than the actual risk.

What Was the State of American Medical Treatment During Puritan Times?

Q: I am working on a report concerning what medical treatment was like in Puritan times. I've searched the Internet for days and can find nothing. Could you help?
Shari Brown
Marietta, Ohio

A: This is obviously a big subject, but in general the sum total of medical knowledge during Puritan times (roughly 1620 until around 1700) was crude, and mostly ineffective. Puritan medicine was wrapped in religion, and there was no scientific basis for any of the treatments offered. The famous Salem witch trials of 1692 were a reflection of how religion controlled so much of Puritan thought. Many diseases were viewed as demonic possession or retribution for some ungodly act.

The social status of the physician in Puritan society was well below that of a member of the clergy, and on a par with a schoolmaster or innkeeper. He had essentially no formal education, and learned what medical care he knew from others in the field. There were no medical schools in the New World. The physician's approach to the patient was also affected by the modesty of the times. For example, examining the chest of a female was not allowed, and as you might imagine, more personal examinations were out of the question. Though the physician would be present, the actual process of childbirth was aided by midwives.

Scientifically speaking, Puritan medicine was not too far removed from that of ancient Greece, in that treatment was more ceremonial than truly medical. Treatments often consisted of casting out demons with spells, chants, and the burning of various substances and inhaling of the smoke. Potions and poultices from plant and animal products were believed to cure a wide variety of ailments. For the most part they didn't. Examples would be things such as Saint-John's-wort to cure madness or to expel demons, and the powder from charred toads for any perceived disease of the blood.

Bloodletting and purging with various diarrhea-inducing plants and minerals were very common. Surgery consisted of cesarean sections, amputations, removing bullets or foreign objects, cleaning and dressing wounds, splinting fractures, and removing stones from the urinary bladder. There were no antibiotics, since the germ theory of disease hadn't even been dreamed of yet. There was no anesthesia. In fact, there was very little that a physician knew or could do. And more often than not he required the blessing of the local clergy before he could do anything.

What Are the Steps Involved in a Psych Evaluation?

Q: I have a character who goes crazy and attacks her boss. The police arrive, take her into custody, and then to the Metropolitan State Hospital in California, where she undergoes a psychological evaluation. What would that involve? The character has a history of emotional tantrums, but can often appear totally normal. Is there a way she could hide her abnormal side during the evaluation? I want her to be held for some time, and then released, so she can stalk the former boss.

Eleanor Thurman
Scottsdale, Arizona

A: There are many standard tests that would be performed to assess her mental abilities. A qualified psychologist or psychiatrist would conduct the examinations and, since this would be a criminal case, a forensic psychiatrist or psychologist would likely be involved. The testing is designed to diagnose any mental disorder, as well as to uncover people who are trying to act crazy or who are trying to hide their mental problems. These tests are mostly subjective, and psychiatrists have been fooled more than once.

The first step would be a complete medical exam to make sure she didn't have some illness or injury that would make her "crazy" or aggressive. Strokes, brain injuries or infections, an overactive thyroid, low blood sugar in diabetics, drug use, and many other things can make someone act very oddly, and at times aggressively. These things must be ruled out before psychiatric testing can be done. To do this she would undergo a complete medical history and physical examination, with special attention to her neurological status. Blood testing, and perhaps specialized brain testing such as an electroencephalogram (EEG) or an MRI or CT brain scan, would follow. If these examinations were normal, the psychiatrist would proceed with his evaluation.

The goal of psychiatric testing would be to determine if she has any significant psychiatric disorders, such as schizophrenia, and to establish her thought processes and cognitive abilities.

Psychiatric testing falls into several categories: personality inventories, projective tests, and intellectual and cognitive assessments. Different psychiatric professionals may employ different tests, but we will consider some of the more common ones.

Personality inventories are designed to determine the subject's basic personality type, and are highly standardized and reliable. Common ones are the Minnesota Multiphasic Personality Inventory (MMPI), the Millon Clinical Multiaxial Inventory (MCMI), and the California Psychological Inventory (CPI). Chances are that you have taken one or more of these tests at some time during your schooling.

Projective tests are designed to evaluate the person's personality and thought processes. They are less standardized and more subjective than the above-mentioned inventories. Common ones include: the Rorschach test, projective drawing, and the Thematic Apperception Test (TAT).

The Rorschach test is the famous inkblot exam. She would be asked to view a series of abstract inkblots and to describe what she sees. How she describes the images may reveal something about her personality, thought processes, and her connection to reality. It may also offer a clue to her inner fantasies.

Projective drawing is similar, except that the subject produces the drawings, which are then analyzed. Your character might be asked to draw a house, a car, a tree, a member of the opposite sex, or a frightening scene or situation. Her drawings may reveal her inner thought processes and her fantasies. For example, if she draws an image of a house that is on fire, a woman who has been stabbed, or a leafless tree with broken branches, these constructs may provide a look into her inner world.

In the Thematic Apperception Test (TAT) she will be shown pictures of common situations and asked to make up a story to go with them. Again, her inner thoughts and fantasies may be revealed. For example, she may be shown a photo of a man and a woman talking. She might then relate a tale of how the two are planning their wedding, or say that they are arguing over money, or that they are saying negative things about her. Obviously, each of these answers would indicate a different psychiatric state.

Intellectual and cognitive testing is designed to assess the subject's intelligence, mental competency, thought processes, and ability to understand their own behavior. The most common intelligence test is the Wechsler Adult Intelligence Scale (WAIS), which would determine her intelligence quotient (IQ).

After these standard tests are completed and evaluated, the psychiatrist will interview the subject. During the interview he will probe deeper into any areas of concern uncovered by the testing process. This is where all his training and experience come into play. Because of the complexity and range of these interviews, and because different psychiatrists use different interview techniques, a complete discussion of this subject here would become a textbook.

However, two interview techniques deserve mention: hypnosis and the use of drugs during the interview process. Hypnosis is used to help suspects and witnesses recall certain events and details. One problem is that it is not very difficult to fake hypnosis, so any information obtained by this technique needs corroboration. Also, persons who are under the influence of hypnosis are often highly suggestible, so that the mere asking of questions may alter their memory of certain events. It is possible that these "new memories" will become part of their "real memory," thus making the validity of any future interviews and court testimony suspect. Some courts allow testimony from previously hypnotized witnesses, others do not.

Though there is no such thing as a "truth serum," certain drugs may lower inhibitions and defenses. Sodium pentothal, the classic truth serum, and other narcotic drugs make the recipient drowsy and euphoric, maybe even chatty. As with hypnosis, any information gleaned in this fashion is suspect, and would likely be challenged in court.

Based on the testing and interview results, the psychiatrist will offer an opinion as to her psychiatric state, competence, and sanity.

He could say whether she had a mental illness or not. He could say whether she was faking or not. It's your call. Either way works, so make the results of the testing or the opinion of the examiner fit your story needs.

What Causes a Person to Become Delusional?

Q: I want my character to become delusional, but I don't want him to have any external signs of illness or injury. In other words, I want him to appear normal. What illness or injury could cause this? I thought Lyme disease might work. Would it? Or can you suggest something else?

Simon Wood
El Sobrante, California
Author of *Working Stiffs* and *Accidents Waiting to Happen*
www.simonwood.net

A: A delusion is a misconception in that the person believes something is true when it is not. He may believe that his neighbor is trying to kill him or that the FBI is tapping his phone. Each of these would be a paranoid delusion. Unless they were true, that is. Or he might believe that he is going to win the lottery or is descended from royalty. These would be delusions of grandeur.

Delusional people maintain contact with reality, unlike people suffering from a psychosis, when contact with reality is lost. The psychotic individual might believe he is Napoléon and is in France in 1803, or that he is Jesus Christ, or that he is a magnificent bird and can fly out of a window. Psychoses are often coupled with hallucinations. This is where someone senses—sees, hears, smells, feels, or tastes—something that is not there. He could see bugs crawling up the wall or the umbrella a man is carrying as a machine gun.

Delusions are psychiatric in origin, so in and of themselves they have no visible physical signs. The defect that causes some delusions may have physical signs, but not the delusion itself. With the exception of delusional thinking the person may act, speak, and interact with others in a normal fashion.

So what causes delusions? Let's look at four categories: psychiatric disorders, diseases, injuries, and drugs.

Many psychiatric diseases have delusions as part of their complex. Schizophrenia is a common one. Schizophrenics may be psychotic or merely delusional. The delusions may be paranoid or fall in one of the many other categories. The victim may appear "crazy" or may behave and appear quite normal. They just have this little psychiatric misunderstanding. It's all a matter of degree. Sufferers of any of the stress disorders such as post-traumatic stress disorder (PTSD) may also have delusions. Your character could have mild schizophrenia or PTSD, and suffer from delusional thinking, yet act and appear normal.

Diseases such as Alzheimer's, senile dementia, multiple-stroke syndrome (someone who has had a number of strokes), marked hyperthyroidism (very overactive thyroid gland), and a number of other problems could cause delusions. Meningitis and other infections of the brain could do the same. Lyme disease, which is an infection contracted through a tick bite, can cause delusions, and even psychoses. An outward manifestation of this latter disease would be a skin rash.

Injuries to the brain may lead to delusions; the classic is a chronic subdural hematoma. This may be what you're looking for in your character. A blow to the head (car accident, fall, or assault) could cause a bleed into the skull but outside the brain. A hematoma (blood clot) then develops between the skull and the brain and can apply pressure to the brain, causing brain dysfunction. The victim may develop headaches, blurred vision, nausea, weakness on one side, and delusions or psychoses. The trauma may be relatively minor, and the hematoma may be delayed for days, weeks, or months. For example, your character could suffer a blow to the head, and several weeks later begin to develop headaches and paranoid delusions. People close to him might notice that his behavior has changed. These changes may be subtle, and outwardly he would appear normal.

Drugs are notorious for causing psychoses and delusions. Cocaine, amphetamines, and heroin use or withdrawal after long-term use may cause delusions, particularly the paranoid types. Delusions and psychoses of various types are very common in chronic alcohol use, and particularly during alcohol withdrawal. Delirium tremens (DTs) is commonly associated with delusions and hallucinations.

Any of these might work for your character.

Can a Brain Injury or Psychological Shock Cause a Temporary Loss of Speech and Hearing?

Q: Can a brain injury and/or psychological trauma induce a temporary loss of hearing and speech? I intend the heroine to regain full possession of her faculties at the end of the story.

Doug Thompson
Niagara Falls, Ontario, Canada

A: The brain is a funny thing, and when it malfunctions almost anything can happen. This means that your scenario can work. With traumatic injuries, some infections, and certain tumors of the brain, various areas of the brain can be damaged, either permanently or temporarily. When this happens, whatever functions that area of the brain controls can fail. This could cause a weakness of one arm or leg, a paralysis of one side of the face, and, if the areas responsible for hearing and/or speech are affected, a loss of these functions. This loss could be permanent or temporary, and if the latter, the problem could last for minutes, hours, days, weeks, months, or years, and then she could return partially or completely to normal. As the injury or infection heals, and if a tumor is successfully removed, complete recovery is possible.

With psychological trauma the same thing could happen. One such scenario is that the person could develop what is called a hysterical conversion reaction. Here the psychological trauma causes the victim to shut down certain brain functions. She may become partially or completely paralyzed, blind, deaf, speechless, or cata-tonic (sits and stares and says nothing nor responds to anyone). A catatonic reaction is the most common form of hysterical conver-sion. With appropriate psychotherapy, conversion reactions can be cured most of the time. This can take days, weeks, months, or years, and more often than not the victim returns to normal.

What Actions Can a Victim of Catatonia Perform?

Q: I am working on a story where one of the characters is catatonic. What causes someone to slip into a catatonic state? What can they do? Walk, eat, talk, move their arms and legs, blink? How would they act? How would a hospital treat them, and what would bring them out of the catatonic state?

A: Catatonia is a psychological condition in which the victim interacts very little with the environment. The victim still hears, sees, and feels, he simply does not respond. He would react to pain, and maybe to an overt threat. Or not. It would depend upon the severity of the condition. True catatonia is not common, but it does occur in some cases of schizophrenia and a few other psychi-atric conditions. Rarely a severe acute trauma, physical or psychi-atric, will trigger a catatonic episode. It may last hours, months, or years. Treatment consists of psychiatric medications and psy-chotherapy. It is often resistant to treatment, and may be difficult to resolve.

The catatonic person tends to sit or lie in one position for long periods. Yes, they blink and may roll over, move to another chair, walk, feed themselves, and do other things. Or they may do almost nothing and their care would fall to someone else. When they move they tend to do so very slowly. They are typically expres-sionless and simply stare at one object or in one direction for long periods. They may or may not look at someone who is speaking to them, and may or may not respond to questions. If they speak it is usually soft, slow, and devoid of emotion or feeling.

Catatonics can do anything; they just often don't. They can feed, dress, and clean themselves. They can walk and talk. Remember, this is a psychiatric condition, not a physical one, so all their abilities exist; they just don't use them.

Your character could have any level of catatonia, and it could last any period of time you wish. This gives you many choices in plotting your story.

What Happens Mentally to Someone Isolated for Long Periods in a Completely Dark Room?

Q: Our hero is going to be locked in a cold, dark basement of an old insane asylum. Since he regularly works with little sleep, he will be tired going in. Given that, how long would it take for him to start questioning his own thoughts, memories, and even what his eyes are seeing (or not seeing) in the total darkness? And once out, would he gain a sense of reality/space/time immediately, or might it take a day, or longer?

P. J. Parrish
Author of *An Unquiet Grave* (a Louis Kincaid mystery)
www.pjparrish.com

A: What you describe is called Sensory Deprivation Syndrome. When placed in an environment devoid of or limited in sensory input, the human mind fills in the blanks. The brain will create sensations, alter sensations, or both. It may construct these sensations from memories, which may indeed be distorted, or may create them from whole cloth. Anyone in such a situation is basically confined to living within his own mind, and the mind is capable of essentially any construct.

In the dark your character might see things such as colors, amorphous objects, floating images, faces, horrible creatures, and virtually anything else his mind could conjure. If quiet, he might hear voices (calling to him, talking about him, or even whispering or singing), bells ringing, scratching or scurrying sounds, growls, and anything else. He might also feel things like cool or warm breezes, bugs crawling on his skin, snakes slithering over his feet and legs, and anything else his mind can construct. And the senses of taste and smell might play a role. He could smell a foul or sweet odor, or perhaps some odor from the past, which could trigger memories, both real and imagined. Smell, the most primitive of our senses, often dredges up memories, frequently of a very visceral nature.

His sensory experiences would not all arise within his own mind. Ambient noises may serve as the seed, and his deprived mind can expand or alter these senses in any direction—good, bad, or just different. For example, he might hear the wind moving a tree branch against the outside wall and think someone or something is digging after him. To save him, to kill him, or to eat him alive. He may hear the screams of other patients far in the distance, and believe they are howling demons coming to take him to hell or angels marching to save his soul. He may feel drips of water or real bugs and conjure a mental army of horrible creatures bent on devouring him.

In the dark his sense of time and place would be severely distorted, and this would only add to his confusion and fuel his imagination further, as would hypothermia (low body temperature) from prolonged exposure to the coldness of the room. People who are hypothermic often develop delusions and hallucinations.

How long would this take? It is widely variable. People react differently to sensory deprivation. Some may be in trouble after only a few hours, while others may require weeks. And anywhere in between.

Once rescued he might recover completely, be left totally insane, or once again anywhere in between. He can recover in an hour or two, a day or two, a month or two, or not at all. Any of these is possible.

This means that you literally have an unlimited array of possibilities. He can sense anything and everything. Whatever you can dream, he can dream. Whatever you can conjure, he can conjure. Any nightmare you can create for him is possible.

Spooky stuff.

What Causes Rage in an Otherwise Normal Person?

Q: I have a character who seems "normal" most of the time, but little things cause episodes of violent anger that are out of proportion to the triggering event. Is there a physical or psychological illness that I could use to account for this? I was thinking of using a compulsive-obsessive type of thing. Would that work?

A: This is a very broad subject that spills over into many medical disciplines, so I'll concentrate on a few conditions that might work for your story.

You alluded to obsessive-compulsive disorder (OCD), which is common and could lead to anger management difficulties. Many people with OCD have minor obsessions, while in others the obsessive behavior controls many of their daily activities. Jack Nicholson played an OCD victim to perfection in *As Good As It Gets*. Most people with OCD have little problem with day-to-day life and tend to "play well with others." But sometimes the need for control, order, and discipline can lead to intolerance of and anger toward others. This may erupt into unexpected outbursts of violent behavior.

Senile dementia and Alzheimer's can lead to anger and acting out. As memory and other brain functions decline, a sense of despair and desperation can grow within the sufferer. This coupled with a decline in cognitive function and a diminished ability to reason can lead to outbursts of anger and violence.

Brain tumors of various types can cause a wide range of psychiatric symptoms, including anger, rage, paranoid ideas, hallucinations, and delusions. These can lead to feelings of persecution or the belief that someone or something is out to get them. These scrambled thought processes might lead to aggressive behaviors, if for no other reason than the perceived need for self-protection. Charles Whitman, the sniper who killed fourteen people from the tower at the University of Texas in 1966, had a small brain tumor.

It may or may not have played a role in his violent behavior, but some tumors in some people definitely do.

Paranoid schizophrenia may lead to similar thoughts and beliefs and result in extremely violent behavior. Remember, to these individuals a perceived threat is a real threat. In fact, it's that way with all of us. But people with schizophrenia don't process information in a normal fashion, and a schizophrenic with a paranoid component to his disease can believe that the people next door are after him, spying on him, or may even have implanted a listening device in his head. To the true paranoid person, attacking or killing the neighbors is a matter of survival. Of course, most individuals with this degree of derangement would not act completely normal at other times. But they might not be stark raving crazy either.

Hypoglycemia can lead to some bizarre behavior, but rarely to violent actions. The brain needs a constant supply of sugar and other nutrients, which it extracts from the blood. Hypoglycemia means a low sugar level in the blood. Symptoms of hypoglycemia are many and varied; common ones are lethargy, hunger, nervousness, anxiety, nausea, fatigue, weakness, dizziness, and personality and psychiatric alterations. Just like some people are mean drunks, others become angry or irritable when they don't eat. Hypoglycemia results when food intake is curtailed, as in crash or fad diets. Also, after a sugary meal or snack, the pancreas releases extra insulin to deal with the sugar load. Often it will release more than is needed, and after the sugar is metabolized (broken down and converted to energy or fat), the excess insulin will rapidly drive the blood sugar down to very low levels. The symptoms of hypoglycemia then follow quickly.

Many drugs can cause anger. Cocaine, methamphetamine, diet pills of various types, and other uppers are notorious for causing anger and paranoia. Withdrawal from narcotics and alcohol can do the same.

Certain seizures can cause aggressive behavior. A seizure is caused when a portion or all of the brain rapidly discharges electrical impulses. The classic grand mal seizure occurs when the entire cortex of the brain is involved. The victim loses consciousness, falls, and displays the classic tonicoclonic jerking motions of the entire body. But some seizures are localized, and their manifestation depends upon which area of the brain is involved. For example, a seizure may be localized to the right arm. It will jerk, while the rest of the body is quiet and the person remains conscious. In this case the seizure focus would be in the left parietal lobe of the brain, in the area that controls the right arm. This type of seizure may remain localized, or it may spread to involve the entire cortex and evolve into a full grand mal seizure.

One type of localized seizure, temporal lobe epilepsy, may be what you need. The temporal lobes of the brain lie in the areas of the brain near the ears. The amygdala is part of the temporal lobe and is involved in emotions, including anger and fear. A seizure confined to this area would have no physical manifestations, such as jerking or loss of consciousness, but rather could cause changes in mood and personality. Anger and rage may result. Or the victim may do things that they ordinarily wouldn't, and have no memory of what they did or where they were. These periods of seizure are called "fugue states." They may last for many hours. The victim can behave in any fashion you want; he can become entirely different from how he is normally. And he may have absolutely no memory of where he went or what he did while the seizure was occurring. He may suddenly wake up and find himself lost or in an odd place or situation. This waking up coincides with the cessation of the seizure activity. Between the seizure episodes the victim would be normal in every way, but during the seizure he could act in any way you want and have absolutely no memory of what happened or what he did.

When I was a medical resident I once saw a young woman who left work for lunch at noon and returned at about 4:30 P.M. When her coworkers asked where she had been, she didn't understand what they were talking about. When she discovered that it was 4:30 and not 1:00 as she'd thought, she freaked. She had no memory of what she had done between leaving her office and returning. Her evaluation revealed that she had temporal lobe epilepsy, and had likely had an episode with a fugue state.

Michael Crichton used this type of seizure in his book *The Terminal Man*.

Any of these could work for your character.

How Was Syphilis Diagnosed and Treated in the 1960s?

Q: I am writing a story set in the late 1950s to early 1960s. My female character has contracted syphilis from her unfaithful husband. How would it have been diagnosed and treated at that time? Did they use antibiotics as standard treatment? If it went undiagnosed for three months, what symptoms would have been prevalent and what would the prognosis have been? Would they have tried to track down the husband (who in the story so far has disappeared without a trace)?

> Michele Cashmore
> Brisbane, Australia
> Author of "The Blank Page," in *Devil in Brisbane*, and
> "Belladonna" in *SF-Envision.com* magazine

A: Syphilis often has no early signs of infection. The classic lesion is a small, nonpainful genital lump or nodule called a "chancre." This chancre is usually a single lesion but at times there can be multiple ones. It appears on the penis or the labia anywhere from a few days to three months after exposure. Or it might not appear at all, or it could be so small that she might ignore it. It goes away three to six weeks after its appearance. This is called primary syphilis. If untreated the disease will progress to the next stage.

Secondary syphilis can occur as the chancre is going away or up to several weeks after. It is characterized by a red or reddish-brown rash that often appears on the palms of the hands and the soles of the feet, but can be anywhere. The person may also develop fever, swollen glands in the neck, sore throat, weight loss, headaches, patchy hair loss, muscle aches, and fatigue. This may last several days or weeks. Again, if untreated it will progress to tertiary syphilis.

Tertiary syphilis begins when the rash disappears. The infection is still in the body, but there are few symptoms and no outward signs of the disease. It progressively damages the brain, heart, major blood vessels in the chest, the liver, the eyes, and the bones and joints. Problems may appear a year later, or up to several decades later. It is very variable.

Your character would not reach the tertiary stage in only three months, but could easily develop some or all of the signs and symptoms of primary and secondary syphilis. Or she could have no symptoms at all and the disease could be diagnosed with a blood test.

At that time the major blood test for syphilis was the VDRL; it took only a few hours to perform. Since syphilis was common, and most people exposed to it did not know they had it, most U.S. states required that this test be performed on all patients admitted to a hospital. Treatment was with high doses of penicillin. Usually an adult would receive 2.4 million units of Bicillin (a type of penicillin) intramuscularly (IM). This was often repeated a week later. The cure rate with this regimen was very high.

The public health services would do whatever they could to locate her estranged husband and anyone else she had had sexual contact with.

When Did Home Pregnancy Testing First Become Available?

Q: My story is set in 1980 and involves home pregnancy testing. Was it available then, and if so, how did it work?
    Catriona Troth
    United Kingdom

A: The first home test was the Early Pregnancy Test, or EPT, and was made by Warner Chilcott. It reached consumers in the late 1970s, so it was around during the time period of your story. It used sheeps' red blood cells (RBCs), which would react with human chorionic gonadotropin (HCG), which is found in the urine of pregnant women and in women with some ovarian tumors. This is an antigen–antibody reaction, and is called a precipitin test. When HCG and sheep RBCs come into contact with one another, they react to form a complex that is not soluble in water (or urine). The newly formed complex will precipitate (become a solid) and drop to the bottom of the testing tube. It can be seen as a ring or clump in the bottom of the tube.

Your young lady would collect a sample of her early morning urine and put a small amount into the EPT testing tube and wait about two hours for the reaction to take place. A positive test would be a white ring of material at the bottom of the tube.

What Injury or Illness Could Prevent My Character from Becoming Pregnant?

Q: My heroine is a thirty-three-year-old ob-gyn physician who has been unable to have children. I need to give her a good reason, recently discovered or occurred, that doesn't involve any potentially fatal diseases (i.e., HIV, ovarian cancer) or a prior pregnancy or venereal disease. And it needs to be an irreversible situation. Maybe some uterine abnormality from birth that was recently discovered or an emergency hysterectomy? Possibly a major auto accident, except that I don't want her to have other physical problems. This discovery or event causes the breakup of her engagement.

Jacqueline Diamond
Brea, California
Author of *A Family at Last* and *Dad by Default*
www.jacquelinediamond.com

A: You have ruled out many common causes of infertility, but there are others.

First of all, some women cannot conceive and the reasons are never discoverable. That is, all anatomic and hormonal tests are normal, yet pregnancy simply will not occur.

Another situation would be that she could suffer from severe uterine fibroid disease. Fibroids are simply masses of benign muscular tumors that grow within the uterus, deforming its shape, and this alteration may prevent pregnancy by preventing implantation of the fertilized zygote into the uterine lining. Fibroids can often lead to severe bouts of pain and bleeding, and at times a complete hysterectomy is the only way to control the problem. This is not uncommon. Your character could suffer from recurrent episodes of abdominal pain with bleeding, and might develop anemia, which would make her weak and short of breath with activity. She would be treated with pain meds and iron, or even a transfusion or two. But if the problem continued, and if the fibroids were too large or too numerous to simply be removed and the uterus preserved, a total hysterectomy would be needed.

Any trauma such as an auto accident could damage the uterus and require its removal. She could suffer this with few other injuries, or at least none that severely limited her in the future. This can happen with seat belt injuries, where the uterine injury could be in conjunction with a bladder rupture. The uterus could be removed in surgery, and the bladder repaired, and she would do well after healing.

Another problem is what is called ovarian failure. Here the ovaries don't produce enough of the hormones needed to support pregnancy, and the victim will be infertile. Blood testing would reveal low levels of hormones such as follicle stimulating hormone (FSH) and luteinizing hormone (LH). She would be otherwise normal, just unable to get pregnant.

What Is the Cause of Death from a Defibrillator Shock?

Q: For my story I'm looking for an unusual weapon for murder. I remember reading somewhere that a cardiac defibrillator can cause death if used improperly. True? How does this work?

A: Yes, a defibrillator can cause death. These devices apply an electric current through the chest to the heart in order to treat both lethal and nonlethal cardiac arrhythmias (changes in heart rhythm). Nonlethal ones tend to come from the atria, the heart's upper chambers. Typical ones would be atrial tachycardia, atrial flutter, and atrial fibrillation. A properly applied electrical current can revert many of these to a normal rhythm. We call this reversion to a normal rhythm "cardioversion."

More lethal rhythms tend to arise from the ventricles, the heart's lower chambers. These would be ventricular tachycardia and ventricular fibrillation. These are the ones that occur in a cardiac arrest, and lead to death in a minute or two unless treated. The use of a defibrillator for electrical cardioversion of these rhythms to a normal rhythm can be life saving.

But one of the more benign atrial rhythms, or even a normal rhythm, can be changed into a deadly ventricular rhythm by an electric shock. This is often what kills people who die from an electric jolt such as that from a live wire, a lightning strike, a wall socket, or a knife stuck into a toaster to retrieve a stuck piece of toast. Yes, your toaster can kill you. People often act without thinking.

The beating of the heart depends upon a rhythmic flow of electricity through it. An electric shock can disrupt this smooth, rhythmic flow and lead to electrical instability, which can lead to dangerous ventricular arrhythmias and death. This means that a defibrillator can be used as a murder weapon. It requires placing electrodes (gel-filled patches) on the victim's chest, connecting the wires from the patches to the defibrillator, charging the defibrillator (takes a few seconds), and then pressing the discharge button. This sends a jolt of electricity into the chest and the heart, and may indeed cause a deadly rhythm. Or it could do nothing except hurt. An electrical current doesn't always kill. Your villain may have to charge the device and repeat the shock.

How Was Diphtheria Treated in 1886 in the American Midwest?

Q: My novel takes place in the American Midwest in 1886. One of my characters comes down with diphtheria, and a young doctor must save her life by employing the latest medical treatments. I believe tracheotomies were performed in those days when the lesion in the throat grew to the point of blocking the windpipe. But when did they begin using intubation? What is the difference between the two?

A: Diphtheria has been recognized for many centuries, and was known to both Muslim and Hebrew physicians many millennia ago. In the Talmud it is referred to as *askara* or *serunke,* and was so feared that as soon as a case appeared within a community a general alarm was sounded by a warning blared from the *shofar,* a ram's horn. Hippocrates gave the first description of the disease in the fourth century B.C. To the ancient Greeks it was *ulcera Syriaca,* and in some Byzantine writings it is termed *esquinancie.* Epidemics periodically ravaged the ancient world and Europe throughout the Dark Ages, Middle Ages, and Renaissance. In the first part of the twentieth century it was a major killer in the United States. In the 1920s, 150,000 cases with 13,000 deaths were reported annually.

Diphtheria is an infectious disease caused by a bacterium called *Corynebacterium diphtheriae.* It infects the pharynx and throat and produces a toxin that can attack the nervous system and damage the heart. In the throat it causes the formation of a thick "scab" called a pseudomembrane. This membrane can peel away from the lining of the throat and obstruct the airway, causing death from asphyxia. The treatment is to establish an "alternate route" for the air to reach the lungs. The first of these was the performance of a tracheotomy—*tracheo* means trachea or windpipe, and *otomy* means to open or create a pathway. Thus, a tracheotomy is the creation of an opening or passageway in the trachea. This is typically done in the front of the throat, just beneath the larynx (voice box or Adam's apple). In this way air can reach the lungs without passing through the throat. In diphtheria, where the pseudomembrane has obstructed the throat, this procedure is life saving.

The first successful tracheotomy was performed on a victim of croup (a disease that can also obstruct the airway) by the French physician Pierre Bretonneau (1771–1862) in Tours on July 1, 1825. He recognized the usefulness of the procedure in diphtheria also.

Interestingly, he is also credited with writing a paper in 1826 in which he gave diphtheria its modern name.

In 1888, Émile Roux and Alexandre Yersin found the diphtheria toxin in cultures of *C. diphtheriae* and two years later, Emil von Behring (1854–1917) used this knowledge, along with knowledge gained from the experiments of Louis Pasteur, and injected attenuated (weakened) diphtheria toxins into guinea pigs, thus making them immune to the disease. He also showed that the serum from the creatures would pass this immunity onto other animals when it was injected into them. A human vaccine for immunization followed.

It was found that many people had an acquired immunity to diphtheria, while others did not. Those who did simply had had contact with the bacterium, and did not become ill, but rather manufactured antibodies to it and were thus immune. In 1913 Béla Schick devised a method (now known as the Schick test) for testing an individual's susceptibility to diphtheria, so that nonimmune persons could be immunized. It was not until the 1930s and 1940s that antibiotics such as penicillin were shown to eradicate the causative bacterium effectively. However, immunization programs became standard for all school children, and soon diphtheria in the United States became a very rare occurrence. By the 1970s fewer than two hundred cases a year were reported.

Endotracheal intubation is the passage of a tube or airway through the mouth or nose and into the trachea to produce a passageway for air to reach the lungs. It is used to support ventilation in patients too weak, ill, or comatose to breathe on their own; to open an airway in persons with head or throat trauma; and in those with airway obstructions from things such as diphtheria. The first intubation was performed by Friedrich Trendelenburg in 1869. He performed the passage of the tube through a tracheotomy opening, however. It was not until about 1900 that intubation of the trachea via the throat or the nose was performed routinely.

Since in 1886 endotracheal intubation would not have been known by your doctor, he could perform a tracheotomy by using a knife to cut through the skin and the trachea in the front of the victim's neck just beneath the Adam's apple. He might cut out a small circle of skin and trachea. There would be pain, of course, and some bleeding. The victim would be able to breathe, the acute illness would resolve over the next week, the tracheotomy wound would gradually close after about three or four weeks, and the victim would go on with life. Your young doctor would indeed be a hero.

Can Exposure to Peanuts Kill Someone Who Is Allergic to Them?

Q: One of my characters attempts to kill a man who is allergic to peanuts by adding them to his food. What symptoms would the victim exhibit? What would the medical examiner find at autopsy?

> **Glenn Ickler**
> **Hopedale, Massachusetts**
> **Author of** Camping on Deadly Grounds **and** Stage Fright

A: The process you are describing is known as acute anaphylaxis, which is a rapid and profound allergic reaction to some antigen. These antigens are typically foods, drugs, or insect venoms. Common foods are peanuts and shellfish; common drugs are penicillin and iodine, which is found in many radiographic dyes; and common insects include bees and wasps. There are myriad other foods, drugs, and bugs that can cause anaphylaxis in the allergic person.

Anaphylaxis is a rapid immune or allergic reaction that involves antigens (the food, drug, etc.) and antibodies, which are manufactured by the body and react to the specific antigen that they are directed against. This reaction is a critical part of our defense against bacteria and viruses. The body recognizes the antigen (a virus, let's say) as foreign, and builds antibodies that will recognize and attach to the virus. This reaction attracts white blood cells (WBCs), which release chemicals that kill or harm the virus, which is then consumed by the WBCs and destroyed. This process is essential for each of us to survive in our bacteria- and virus-filled world.

But in allergic individuals this reaction is rapid and massive, and causes a release of large amounts of the chemicals from the WBCs, and it is these chemicals that create the problems. They cause dilatation (opening up) of the blood vessels, which leads to a drop in blood pressure (BP) and then to shock. They cause the bronchial tubes (airways) to constrict (narrow severely), which leads to shortness of breath, wheezing, and cough. This is basically a severe asthmatic attack, and it prevents adequate air intake, so the oxygen level in the blood drops rapidly. The chemicals also cause what is known as "capillary leak." This means that the microscopic blood vessels in the tissues begin to leak fluids into the tissues, which leads to edema (swelling). In the skin this is manifested as hives and rashes. In the lungs it causes swelling of the airways that along with the constriction of the breathing tubes prevents air intake. In the tissues it causes swelling of the hands, face, eyes, and lips. The net result of an anaphylactic reaction is a dramatic fall in BP, severe wheezing, swelling and hives, shock, respiratory and cardiac failure, and death.

Usually anaphylaxis onsets within minutes (ten to twenty) after contact with the chemical, but sometimes, particularly with ingested foods, it may be delayed for hours—even up to twenty-four hours.

At autopsy the findings are nonspecific. That is, they are not absolutely diagnostic that an anaphylactic reaction occurred. The ME would expect to find swelling of the throat and airways, and perhaps fluid in the lungs (pulmonary edema), and maybe some bleeding in the lungs. He may also find some congestion of the internal organs, such as the liver. He must, however, couple these findings with a history of the individual having eaten a certain food, having ingested or being given a certain drug, or having received an insect bite or sting and then developing symptoms and signs consistent with anaphylaxis. Also, in the case of insects, he may be able to (or not) find antibodies to the insect's venom in the victim's blood, thus proving the bee venom was the antigen that caused the reaction.

In your scenario, if the victim had a severe allergy to peanuts, contact with peanuts or peanut oil could lead to a rapid and severe anaphylactic reaction. Five minutes or even less would be possible. The victim would proceed through the above symptoms and signs, and could die in a very few minutes. The ME could find swelling in the throat and lungs, and might learn from witnesses, police reports, or other sources that the victim had contact with peanuts or peanut oil or some food product containing either of these, and determine that anaphylaxis was the likely cause of death. Or there could be no witnesses and the autopsy could be essentially normal. You can craft your scene either way and it'll work.

I should point out that this method of murder was used in the wildly successful novel *The Da Vinci Code.*

What Problems Could a Physician Have in 1816 That Would Lead to His Being Ostracized by the Medical Community and Society in General?

Q: I'm writing about Napoléon in exile on St. Helena. His doctor at that time was Barry O'Meara. For plot purposes I would like O'Meara to be harboring a secret— perhaps some spectacular medical failure—that has forced his retreat to St. Helena in an attempt to reverse his fortunes. What sort of event could ruin the professional and possibly personal reputation of a doctor in England in 1816?

> Laura Harrington
> Gloucester, Massachusetts
> Playwright of N *(Bonaparte)*
> www.pilgrimtheatre.com

A: There are many possibilities: He could have been incompetent and botched several surgical procedures, or dishonest in his billings, or perhaps failed to save the wife or child of a VIP or government official, or have had a problem with alcohol or opium (a commonly abused substance during that time period). But perhaps— and I like this one—he could have been like Dr. Knox in the infamous case of Burke and Hare that occurred around the same time period. Burke and Hare procured bodies for Dr. Knox's dissection demonstrations, which were used to teach other doctors. They began by digging up fresh corpses, for which they received six pounds per body in summer and ten in winter. (I guess it was more difficult to rob graves when the ground was cold.)

But the local populace was uncooperative and refused to die fast enough for the greedy men. To get around this little bump in the road they simply began kidnapping people who were not likely to be missed and killing them. Burke, who was a large man, would sit on them and hold their mouth and nose closed until they suffocated. This technique became known as "Burking." Over the next year, sixteen people met such a fate.

A lodger at the hotel notified authorities when she discovered their sixteenth and last victim beneath a bed. Apparently the two men had stashed the body there while awaiting an opportunity to transport it to Surgeons Square, where Dr. Knox performed his dissections. The two men were arrested. Hare then turned king's evidence on Burke, and testified against him. Burke was convicted and hanged on January 28, 1829, an event attended by as many as forty thousand people.

Your doctor could have lied about his involvement in such a grave robbing and/or murder scheme, and perhaps there wasn't enough evidence to show that he knew where the bodies came from, so he was never tried. However, the public outcry or a snubbing by his professional colleagues could have resulted in his being run out of town for his role in the activities. He could have fled to St. Helena, where he came to care for Bonaparte.

How does that work for you?

What Traumatic Injury Can Recur and Become Life Threatening a Year Later?

Q: I have a protagonist who must sustain injuries in the crash of a corporate jet in which he is the sole survivor. He recovers in a few months and then, about a year later, the injury or condition needs to result in a life-

threatening relapse that comes on suddenly, requiring
hospitalization in the ICU. Any suggestions?

A: Your best bet is a delayed or recurrent dissection of the aorta.
Let me explain.

The aorta is the main artery from the heart to the body. All the
blood pumped from the heart passes into the aorta, which arcs up
and to the left, giving off branches to the right arm (right subclavian artery), the right and left carotids (arteries on both sides of the
neck that supply the brain), and the left arm (left subclavian
artery), and then continues downward along the back of the chest
and the abdomen, where it divides into branches to each leg (right
and left iliac arteries). As you can see, the aorta is very important.

In severe trauma, such as automobile accidents, falls, plane
crashes, and other bad stuff, the aorta can tear or rupture and bleed,
leading to almost instantaneous death. But sometimes it is only
partially torn. Here, rather than a sudden collapse and death, the
victim would experience severe chest and back pain and shortness
of breath, which could be construed as part and parcel of the
trauma rather than the serious medical condition that it truly is. In
this case it can rupture at a later time, such as hours, days, or weeks
later, or it can heal and life goes on. So far so good.

Rarely, such an injury can heal, and then years later dissect (tear)
again. This can result from another trauma, more minor this time;
from long-standing untreated hypertension (high blood pressure);
or from bad luck. Again the symptoms are chest and back pain and
shortness of breath. The treatment is immediate hospitalization in
an ICU and the administration of pain medications (morphine or
Demerol) and meds that lower the blood pressure (beta blockers
such as Inderal or Tenormin or other BP-lowering drugs, such as
nitroprusside, which is given by intravenous [IV] drip). The lowering of the blood pressure is to lessen the pressure on the aorta, and
thus hopefully slow the dissection and stabilize the victim enough
to get him into surgery alive. The victim is then taken to the operating room (OR), where a cardiovascular surgeon repairs or
replaces the aorta with a graft of Dacron or a similar material.

Major surgery, but if the victim survives and gets through a few months of healing, he'll do well.

In your scenario the executive could suffer chest trauma, maybe a broken rib or two, and an undiagnosed aortic dissection (these are easy to miss). He would be banged up for from several weeks to a couple of months, and then would feel okay. Only later would he develop severe, tearing pain in his chest and upper back. He would go to the hospital, where a chest X-ray would show a widened aortic shadow. This simply means that the area of the X-ray where the aorta is visible is wider than usual, which is from the tear. An MRI would be done, an aortic dissection would be diagnosed, and the patient would head off to the OR.

Could Death from a Pulmonary Embolus Follow a Severe Beating?

Q: My character is a twenty-year-old man who is thin, and in good shape and good health. He is attacked, severely beaten, and loses consciousness after receiving a head injury and a broken arm. It is fourteen to sixteen hours before he receives medical attention. While waiting for help, I want him to suffer a pulmonary embolism along with his other ailments. Is this scenario plausible? What kind of injuries would cause an embolism?

> Ginger Robinson
> Master of Fine Arts student

A: An embolus is the generic term for any object that travels through the bloodstream and lodges somewhere. A pulmonary embolus (or PE, for short) is a blood clot that travels through the right side of the heart and lodges in the lungs. The clots responsible for this most often form in the large veins of the pelvis and the legs, and very rarely in the veins of the arms. Overweight and elderly persons are more prone to them, in general, but the conditions that truly promote the formation of clots and emboli are more related to injuries to the legs and/or pelvis and to immobilization.

Auto accidents, falls, and other traumatic injuries to the legs and pelvis are often accompanied by injuries to the veins in the area, and injured veins tend to clot. Bruises and fractures of the legs or hips are particularly dangerous.

With immobilization the blood tends to stagnate (to a degree) in the immobilized area, and this too promotes clot formation and embolization. Anyone who is ill or injured and must remain in bed for several days becomes prone to emboli.

Surgery is also a risk factor for PE. After surgery people are often required to stay in bed for several days, and this can lead to clots and emboli. This is particularly true if they have had abdominal, hip, or leg surgery.

The problem with your scenario is the nature of the injuries and the timing. First of all, trauma to the arms and head are very unlikely to cause clots and emboli. Legs okay, not arms. Clots usually take several days to form, so these emboli tend to occur several days or weeks after the injury. But not always.

How can you make your scenario work? Use a combination of leg injuries and immobilization. This is a very dangerous situation, and a PE is not uncommon in such cases. Have your character beaten severely about the head to the point that he is in a coma afterward, and thus unmoving. Have him also beaten in the leg area. Maybe he is kicking at his attacker and many of the assailant's blows, either from fists or from some object like a bat or a board, are to the victim's legs, resulting in deep bruises. The victim would then have leg injuries and be immobile for twelve or more hours, and this could lead to clots and emboli, and he could die during the fourteen or so hours before he is found. Or he could be found alive and be taken to a hospital and admitted to the ICU for observation and treatment. After a day or two or more, as you need, he could suffer a sudden cardiac arrest (heart stops) and die. The autopsy could then show he had suffered a massive pulmonary embolus.

Was the Term "Cancer" Known in 1833?

Q: I'm working on a story set in 1833. Was the term "breast cancer" known or used at that time?

Win Blevins

Author of *Give Your Heart to the Hawks* and *Stone Song*

A: Yes. Cancer was recognized in ancient Egypt and was mentioned in the famous Edwin Smith Papyrus. The term "cancer" was coined by Hippocrates in approximately 400 B.C. He called them "carcinomas," a term that is still used today. By the seventeenth and eighteenth centuries many forms of cancer were recognized, including breast cancer. In fact, in 1713 Bernardino Ramazzini postulated that the high incidence of breast cancer in nuns was due to their celibate lifestyle.

How Was Breast Cancer Treated in 1826?

Q: I'm working on a period piece (circa 1826) that includes a woman developing breast cancer. How would a typical case at this time manifest itself? How would a patient know something's wrong, and what would be the typical course of the disease? Was it always fatal? Were any surgical techniques attempted? What treatment (were they still bleeding patients then?) might be given? How would the pain be treated?

A: Breast cancer in 1826 was the same disease as it is now. The symptoms when untreated are: a rapidly growing breast lump that may or may not be painful; swelling of the lymph nodes within the axilla or armpits (these are hard lumps that may also be painful, or not); weakness; weight loss; poor appetite; and symptoms associated with metastatic disease, as noted on the following page (metastatic means that the cancer has spread to somewhere else in the body). Common sites for breast cancer would be:

Brain: She may develop severe headaches, blurred or double vision, nausea and vomiting, perhaps weakness on one side of the body, and ultimately coma and death.

Bones: This cancer often spreads to the ribs and spine, causing a deep, boring, burning pain that is very difficult to relieve, even today with more powerful medications.

Lungs: She might develop sharp chest pains that become worse with breathing, or a cough, and she might cough up some blood. She would be very fatigued and short of breath with almost any activity, and even at rest.

Liver: She could become jaundiced, which is a yellow discoloration of the skin and the whites of her eyes. She could develop right upper abdominal pain, along with nausea, vomiting, and weight loss.

There was no treatment, and no surgery would likely be done. It was essentially 100 percent fatal. Barring miracles. She would be given medications for pain, most likely alcohol or laudanum (tincture of opium). Bloodletting would be possible but would not likely be done for this. It was falling from favor about this time, though it did persist into the twentieth century in some areas.

What Tests or Examinations Can Be Used to Distinguish an Adult of Small Stature from a Child?

Q: One of my adult characters is able to pass herself off as a child due to her short stature and youthful features. Another one of my characters, one with considerable medical experience, must discover her real age and deduce the cause of her shortness, that being a poor diet when she was young. I need to know how he could do this.

INJURIES, ILLNESSES, DOCTORS, AND HOSPITALS

A: Yes, this may be possible. X-rays, particularly of the arms, legs, hands, and skull, can give clues to a person's age. Bones grow and calcify (change from cartilage to bone by the collection of calcium within them) at a predictable rate and in a predictable pattern. This is particularly helpful in determining age before about twelve to fifteen, but can be useful on up to about twenty-five. Also, thinning or loss of minerals in the bones and arthritis in the joints can often reveal that a person is over fifty as compared to twenty or thirty.

Bones grow at the epiphyses (growth plates). These are bands near the ends of our long bones—arms and legs. These areas continually add length until the epiphyses "close"—turn to bone. After this the bones can no longer lengthen. This occurs around age eighteen to twenty. So bones with "open" epiphyses indicate a younger age, while those that are closed suggest an age greater than twenty. Malnutrition may delay this process, and may cause certain deformities, both grossly and microscopically, in the bones. It is complex and difficult to explain, but just know that an X-ray may suggest the presence of malnutrition, particularly during the growth years.

Your character could take, have taken, or find X-rays from the suspect and have a radiologist or anthropologist review them and determine the person's age and earlier nutritional status. Or not. It's not always possible, but if you need this determination for your story it will work.

Could a Young Girl Survive Gangrene and a Leg Amputation in the Western Frontier in the Late 1800s?

Q: In my story a young girl loses her leg to gangrene and amputation during a late 1800s transcontinental trip from the East Coast to the Western frontier. Medical care being what it was during the period, is it possible that she could survive such an ordeal? What exactly would the amputation involve?

Mike Dunn, screenwriter
Orange, California

A: At that time gangrene was fairly common, difficult to treat, and carried a very high mortality rate. Gangrene is a wound infection caused by the bacterium *Claustridium perfringens*. The wound that opens the door for such an infection could be a major injury such as a gunshot wound, or as minor as a puncture from a thorn. Today treatment includes debridement (the surgical removal of any infected tissues) and high doses of antibiotics. During the time period of your story there were no antibiotics, so amputation offered the only effective treatment. If the leg were left attached the infection would enter the bloodstream, and death would be very likely.

Amputations during the nineteenth century were dangerous and brutal. The surgeon attempted to do the procedure as fast as possible since it was very painful, and in frontier areas or during times of war anesthetic agents weren't readily available. The typical anesthetic was either alcohol or tincture of opium, but surely ether was used too. Dr. Crawford Long first employed ether in surgery in Atlanta, Georgia, in 1842, and then later the first public demonstration of it took place in Boston in 1846. So it would be realistic for one of your characters to have access to it, and to have the skills to use it and perform an amputation. Remember, there were few true doctors, and often these things were done by someone in the traveling community. The group leader, the blacksmith, or anyone else could be the "surgeon."

Even with a whiff of ether the patient would likely have to be restrained by some of the stronger members of the community. A tourniquet would be tied around the extremity, and a large knife would be used to cut the tissues circumferentially down to the bone. A handsaw would then be used to cut the bone. The stump would be cauterized (burned) with a hot blade or other piece of metal heated over a fire, and dressed with the cleanest pieces of cloth available.

The mortality rate for these procedures in the late 1800s was 50 percent or more. Usually from infection, though bleeding and shock claimed others. So your young lady's chances would be fifty-fifty at best, but she could definitely survive the ordeal.

What Medical Treatments for Pain and Injury Were Available in Ancient Egypt?

Q: What were the most common medicinal herbs available in Egypt around A.D. 80? I am particularly interested in wound healing/protection and pain-relief medications, preferably topically applied and acceptable to both humans and animals.

    Cathy Fishburn
    Yorba Linda, California

A: As with other ancient civilizations, Egyptian medicine was a combination of spiritual beliefs, social conventions, and empiric observations (learning via trial and error). In addition, they inherited a strong belief in astrology from the Babylonians. Also, as with other ancients, the Egyptians possessed a certain *materia medica*, literally the materials of medicine. These included various potions, oils, salves, and ointments usually derived from plant and animal products. They were often applied and/or taken with great ceremony, which was designed to appease an angry god or attract one with healing powers. Imhotep was the Egyptian god of health and healing, and most incantations were addressed to him. He was actually a mortal who served as vizier under King Zoser, who served during the Third Dynasty until about 2980 B.C. Imhotep was a gifted healer, and was later deified as the god of medicine.

What we know of Egyptian medical treatment predominantly comes from several papyri that were discovered centuries later. These tend to be named for the person who discovered them. The most important are the Kahun Papyrus (c. 1850 B.C.), the Edwin Smith Papyrus (c. 1600 B.C.), the Ebers Papyrus (c. 1550 B.C.), and the London Papyrus (c. 1350 B.C.). Several sections of these treasured documents deal with various medical and surgical issues. For example, the Ebers Papyrus lists seven hundred to eight hundred formulas for the treatment of medical problems.

Myrrh, frankincense, and manna were thought to help heal

wounds and other illnesses. Antimony, copper, and other metals when mixed with various herbs were believed to aid wound healing when used as a cleaning astringent. Animal organs such as pig brain and ox spleen were mixed with animal fat and honey and taken orally or smeared over wounds. Sometimes tortoiseshells or even crushed lapis lazuli was added. Purgatives came from plant extracts made from senna, colocynth, and castor oil. Garlic, onion, tamarisk, honey, opium, cannabis, hellebore, and even animal excrement (crocodile dung held special power) were mixed and applied as ointments and poultices, compacted into pills and swallowed, mixed with liquids for gargling, given as suppositories, or heated and used as fumigants.

Humans and animals received similar treatments for the most part.

Can the Injection of Air into a Vein Cause Death?

Q: I am writing a book in which a young woman is killed by a quantity of air being injected into a vein in her ankle. Would this work? The body is then dumped into the sea (a Scottish estuary in August) but is found after a few hours. Would the coroner think she had drowned or would he be able to determine the true cause of death? Would there be any sign at all of a needle mark?

Kate Atkinson
Edinburgh, United Kingdom
Author of *One Good Turn*

A: The veins around the ankle are called the posterior tibial (behind the lateral or outside ankle bone) and the dorsalis pedis (travels across the top of the foot). These veins join together in the lower calf to produce the popliteal vein, and then travel on up to become the femoral vein in the groin. Air injected into either of these veins will follow this path, and then travel up the inferior vena cava and into the heart.

This bubble of air is called an air embolus. But contrary to popular belief, a small air bubble will not kill a person. And it will not
travel to the brain and cause a stroke. Why? The lungs get in the
way. In order to reach the brain the air must pass through the right
side of the heart, the pulmonary (lung) vessels, through the left side
of the heart, and then up to the brain. The lung would filter out
the bubble, and it would never reach the left side of the heart or the
brain.

To kill, an air embolus must be a bolus (wad or mass) of air
about 100 or so ccs—about half a cup. When injected rapidly this
bolus of air would travel into the right side of the heart and prevent the pumping action of the blood. Blood is a liquid, and is not
compressible. When the right ventricular heart muscle contracts,
the liquid blood is squeezed out and into the lungs. If the right
ventricle is filled with air, the air is compressible and thus will not
be squeezed forward; it will simply be compressed into a smaller
volume and stay where it is, becoming sort of a vapor lock. This
stops blood flow and can lead to cardiac arrest and death in a
minute or two.

Since the body in your scenario is found quickly no decay
would have occurred, so the ME would have an intact corpse to
work with. He would easily determine that the victim did not
drown, and would see a mass of air in the right ventricle and know
that the victim died of an air embolus. He would then search for
and most likely find the injection site.

Can a Corpse Be Bled After Death?

Q: I need to know about blood flow after death. For a
book set in the Middle Ages in Europe I need to have a
young victim die quickly from a sacrificial wound made
with a sharp flint or obsidian knife blade. He is then
bled by someone using a hollow animal bone inserted
into the wound. This is a ritual death and not torture, so
I need to have the victim either already dead or com-

pletely unconscious. Where should the wound be? Will the blood flow after death, and if so, for how long? Or will I have to have the victim remain unconscious?

Richard Devlin
San Francisco, California

A: Blood flow will stop at death. When the heart stops beating, blood flow halts immediately. Any bleeding after death would be oozing and trickling. This would follow the law of gravity, so only wounds on the downside of the body would ooze. For your victim, if he was stabbed with the knife or with the hollow tube in the left side and he was rolled onto his left side, he might trickle and ooze for a few minutes. On the contrary, if he were placed on his right side, with the wound facing up, he would ooze very little if at all. Regardless, the blood would clot in five to ten minutes, and all oozing would stop.

If you need to collect several containers of blood the hollow bone should be inserted while the victim is still alive. Sedation or intoxication would have no effect on the flow of blood unless the victim died from the sedation. The best place to insert the hollow bone would be into a vein. The neck, arm, or groin areas would be best. Or it could be placed through the upper right part of the abdomen where the liver is located. The liver is filled with blood and will bleed when punctured. If the knife wound was in the right upper abdomen and the bone were pushed through it and into the liver while the victim was alive, you could remove a great deal of blood, three or four pints, before he slipped into shock and died from blood loss.

There's nothing quite like old-time religion, is there?

What Are the Physical Findings and Mechanism of Death in a Victim Whose Face Is Held Beneath Boiling Water?

Q: If the victim in my story has his face and head pushed into a large pot of boiling water until dead, what visible injuries would be found on the corpse (especially skin and eyes) if discovered fifteen to thirty minutes after death? What would be the exact mechanism of death in such a case (drowning? the burns? something else?)? Would the finger marks of the murderer be left in some way on the neck/throat of the victim (assuming the murderer held the victim from behind, forcing his face into the boiling water)? Would the victim's body be hot to the touch if the body were found within fifteen minutes of death?

A: The face and any other surfaces that contacted the boiling water would be severely burned and blistered. The burns most likely would be a combination of second and third degree. The skin would be red and raw, and large blisters (called bullae in medical jargon) would be present. There would be areas where the skin completely sloughed off (peeled or burned away). The eyes would be similarly damaged, and the eyelids would be swollen and burned. As the victim breathed in the hot water, the nasal passages, mouth, throat, bronchi (breathing tubes), and lungs would be severely burned and injured.

The cause of death would be drowning. The burns would not kill, and with the killer's hands on the back of the victim's neck strangulation would not likely occur.

Yes, the killer would have to use a great deal of force and effort to hold the victim's face beneath the water, and this would leave strangulationlike bruises on the back and sides of the neck. These bruises would be blue-black in color. I assume that the killer would wear some type of heat-resistant gloves to avoid scalding his own hands, and if so these bruises would be diffuse and indistinct but still might reflect a finger pattern.

The heat of the boiling water on the face would not be transmitted to the body, so the body temperature would be normal and would decline over time, as with any other corpse. This rate is approximately 1 to 1.5 degrees per hour under normal environmental conditions.

How Could a Serial Rapist Be Rendered Impotent by a Drug or a Surgical Procedure in the 1960s?

Q: In our story set in the 1960s a psychiatrist must release a violent rapist into the world but fears he will rape and kill again. We need her to do something to him before his release that will render him impotent or incapable of completing the act. This needs be done surgically or with a one-time drug.

P. J. Parrish
Author of *An Unquiet Grave* (a Louis Kincaid mystery)
www.pjparrish.com

A: The most effective direct thing would be castration. This is a simple and quick surgical procedure in which the scrotum is opened and the testes are removed. This was and still is advocated by some to lower the risk of releasing known serial rapists into the public.

Currently there are drugs that cause a "chemical castration." For the most part these are female hormones that suppress testosterone in these men and hopefully lessen aggression and sex drive, and change the tone of the perpetrators' fantasies to more passive ones. It is controversial but used in several states today. In 1996 California became the first state to pass such laws. Florida, Louisiana, Georgia, Oregon, Montana, Texas, and Wisconsin soon followed. Depo-Provera, which is an injectable drug, is the one typically used.

But these weren't available in the 1960s, and there was no other medication that would fit your needs. Go with castration. That works for your story.

What Injuries Occur After a Fork Stab to the Throat?

Q: One of my characters jams a fork into the throat of another. The attack is from the front, his trachea is punctured, and the fork is left in place. How much bleeding would occur, how badly would his breathing be impaired, how would someone handle such an injury at the scene to try to save the guy's life, and how long could he last without treatment?

David Corbett

Author of *The Devil's Redhead, Done for a Dime,*

and *Blood of Paradise*

www.davidcorbett.com

A: What happens depends upon what structures are injured. A fork or any penetrating object to the throat could damage several things. The carotid arteries, jugular veins, trachea (windpipe), larynx (voice box or Adam's apple), and the thyroid gland could easily be hit.

The carotid arteries (one on each side of the neck in the hollow beside the larynx) carry blood from the aorta to the brain. If either is damaged, severed, or occluded in any way, blood supply to the brain could be curtailed immediately and the victim would likely collapse and die within seconds or minutes. If nicked, the bleeding would be profuse and pulsatile (pumping) in quality, and the victim would bleed out in a few minutes. Until he lost consciousness he could talk or shout.

The jugular veins (one on each side, and they lie very near the carotids) carry blood from the brain to the superior vena cava and on to the heart. If injured as above, the bleeding would be brisk and nonpulsatile, and the victim would not die immediately, since the blood flow to the brain is unaltered. At least until the bleeding was sufficient to drop the blood pressure (BP) and produce shock. At this point the victim would lose consciousness and die from exsanguination (bleeding to death). This could take many minutes, or the bleeding could stop and the victim survive. Either is possible.

The thyroid lies on either side of the trachea, and a portion (called the thyroid isthmus) passes over the trachea to connect the two halves. It is in the area just beneath the larynx. If injured it will bleed severely, but not usually enough to lead to exsanguination. However, if the trachea or larynx is also punctured, blood from the damaged thyroid might enter the trachea and lungs and cause severe breathing difficulties, and even death, from literally drowning in blood.

Injuries to the trachea or larynx are similar, except that the vocal cords lie within the larynx and may be damaged with injury to that area. Thus, speech will be raspy or impossible. A rent or puncture of any significant size in the trachea beneath the larynx will prevent speech or the making of any noise whatsoever. Why? To make noise, any noise, air must pass over the vocal cords. If the hole in the trachea is beneath the larynx, as it essentially always will be, air from the lungs will pass through the hole and out of the body and never reach the vocal cords. With a small hole such as those made with a fork tine, enough air would likely reach the cords to make some noise. The victim could grunt and groan and perhaps whisper, but probably couldn't cry out.

Now to your victim.

A fork to the front of the trachea would likely not damage either the carotids or the jugulars, so sudden death and severe bleeding would not be likely to occur. If the thyroid were punctured some bleeding would be present, and this could be severe or minor, as you need for your scene. Either is possible. His breathing could be severely impaired or only a little so. Again, as you need. Could your victim speak or yell? In your story, probably so, since the fork remains in place. This would effectively plug the holes, and air would then pass along the normal path and past the vocal cords.

The key to treatment is twofold: controlling bleeding and maintaining an open airway so the victim can breathe. Local pressure over the wound may stop or slow the bleeding. If the victim is bleeding into the trachea and lungs, this is a much bigger problem.

Here the victim should be rolled to one side so that blood can more easily drain out through the throat and mouth and, more important, any blood that enters the lungs will by gravity be directed to the lower one—called the dependent one. The lung away from the floor would remain dry and functional. Since only one lung is needed to live, the victim could survive for a long time and be transported to a hospital in this same position. Should the fork be removed? Most likely yes, and especially if it is obstructing the airway. The only time it might be better to leave it would be if it were jammed through a carotid artery or a jugular vein and removing it would lead to more bleeding. This would not be a common situation but could happen.

What Is the Most "Merciful" Way to Kill Someone with a Knife?

Q: Is there such a thing as a "merciful" way to kill someone with a knife? I'm looking for a murder method using a bladed instrument that would be relatively painless and kill instantly. I'd also need to know how much blood loss would be involved in order to accurately describe the crime scene.

> Gar Anthony Haywood (writing as Ray Shannon)
> Los Angeles, California
> Shamus- and Anthony-award-winning author
> of *Man Eater* and *Firecracker*
> www.garanthonyhaywood.com

A: The most merciful use of a knife for murder would be by slipping it between two of the cervical vertebrae (neck spinal bones) and severing the spinal cord. The victim would immediately collapse, since all connection between the brain and the legs and other muscles would be interrupted. The legs and the entire body would be suddenly limp, like a puppet whose strings had been cut. The victim would also lose consciousness due to what is called "spinal shock." When the spinal cord is damaged or transected (cut in half), as would be the case here, the blood vessels of the body immediately dilate (open up) and the blood pressure (BP) drops dramatically. The victim passes out in a matter of seconds, and dies. There would likely be little blood since the wound is small, and when the BP drops very low there is little pressure to cause bleeding. And when the heart stopped in a minute or so, there would be no blood flow and thus no bleeding. Dead folks don't bleed. So maybe a few tablespoons to half a cup at the most. If the knife were left in place for a couple of minutes, until the victim is dead, there would be essentially no external bleeding.

Another possibility would be a slashing of one or both of the carotid arteries. These lie along either side of the trachea (windpipe) and carry blood from the heart to the brain. When cut they will pump a lot of blood—like a geyser. These spurts would gradually diminish in distance and volume as the BP falls, and finally bleeding would stop when the heart stops. This could take a couple of minutes. With the interruption of one or both carotids the victim could lose consciousness immediately, or if not would do so after a minute or two, as he slipped into shock from blood loss.

Can a Condom Be Used to Save the Life of Someone Suffering Severe Lacerations from Shattered Glass?

Q: I'm writing a scene where a physician is in the front office of a dive motel, standing near a condom vending machine, when a car clips the window, shattering it, then is involved in a collision with another car in the street. Is there some clever way he could use the condoms to save the life of someone injured either by the flying glass or by the collision? He then goes with the victim to the local ER. How would he treat minor wounds from flying glass? Would he simply remove the shards with tweezers, disinfect the wounds, and apply bandages?

Lee Goldberg
Los Angeles, California

Author of the Diagnosis Murder and Monk series
www.leegoldberg.com

A: What a cool idea. Yes, this will work.

If a piece of the glass from either the window or the car's wind-shield or windows sliced an artery in the victim's arm or leg, your M.D. could use a condom, or several twisted together, as a tourni-quet. The injured artery could be the radial artery on the thumb side of the wrist, the brachial artery in the bend of the elbow, or the popliteal artery behind the knee. The tourniquet would be placed proximal to (above) the injury and twisted tightly enough to stop the blood flow.

At the hospital the artery would be repaired first, since that is the major injury. This would be done either in the emergency room or the operating room. After this all the other wounds would be cleaned, sutured if necessary, and dressed. Yes, tweezers are used to pick out the pieces of glass, and the wounds would be thoroughly cleaned. Also, X-rays would be taken, since small pieces of glass that may not be readily visible can usually be seen on an X-ray. This way they could be sure that all the pieces were removed. This is often more difficult than it sounds. Those little devils can hide.

He would be admitted to the hospital for a couple of days and given antibiotics to prevent infection, and he should do well, since your physician jumped in and saved the day.

What Type of Injury Could Cause Temporary Paralysis After Which the Victim Would Be Normal?

Q: I am writing a story set in early-nineteenth-century London. Is it possible for my character to survive a blow from a vehicle or a fall that would render him paralyzed from the waist down for a couple of months, after which he would return to normal? Would there be pain or numbness? What methods would be employed to evaluate and treat the condition, and what care of the patient would be necessary? With no X-rays available would it be known that complete recovery was possible from the outset? How would his return to normal manifest? Quickly or over a period of time?

Hazel Statham
Staffordshire, England
Author of *Dominic* and *My Dearest Friend*
www.hazel-statham.co.uk

A: Your scenario works very well.

Any type of trauma to the lower back could lead to paraplegia, which is paralysis from the waist downward. A fall, a horse-cart collision, or a gunshot could each cause this.

He could have a fracture of his lumbar (lower back) vertebrae (spinal column bones), or not. The bones could be intact and the injury could be confined to the muscles and other tissues of the lower back. Regardless, the injury would contuse (bruise) the spinal cord, causing swelling and bleeding in the area. This swelling and the accumulation of blood could put pressure on the spinal cord, which would interfere with its functioning and cause paraplegia. The legs would be limp, paralyzed, and numb. As the swelling resolved—this could take days, weeks, or a couple of months—the first thing he would sense is paresthesia. This is the tingling you feel when your leg "goes to sleep." He would then be able to sense touch. This would at first be a vague sensation but would progressively become more normal day by day. Movement would also begin to return. At first he would be able to wiggle his toes, then move his feet, and then his legs. Soon he would be able to sit, stand, and then walk. This progression may take weeks or months.

There was little treatment available at the time of your story. He would be placed in bed rest and treated with various herbs, which would make absolutely no difference in his recovery. The local doc would come see him, but he could do little. He would not know whether the victim was going to get better or be unable to walk ever again. He may have seen similar injuries that went both ways, and he may say as much. But he wouldn't know for sure.

What Happens in a "Hysterical Pregnancy"?

Q: For a character in my story I need some information about a so-called hysterical pregnancy. How does it manifest? Can the woman go so far as to miss periods and start to show?

A: Hysterical pregnancy is called pseudocyesis. It is a psychiatric disorder and has many manifestations, which vary from person to person and depend upon the severity of the mental illness.

When full blown the sufferer can exhibit the cessation of periods, weight gain, abdominal distention, morning sickness, and all the other symptoms of a real pregnancy. Some will stuff pillows or clothing into their own clothing to appear even more pregnant. Some are very clever, so that the pregnancy "progresses" as expected. They might fake visits to a doctor, and may even go so far as to steal an infant from a hospital, friend, relative, or public place at the time of "delivery." There have even been cases where pregnant women have been murdered and their child cut from their bodies. Some mental disorders have no bounds.

How Was Mental Illness Treated in 1870?

Q: I don't know if you know anything about the history of sedatives, but I'm finding it especially difficult to research. My story takes place in a London asylum circa 1870. What treatments were used during that era? What would be used to sedate a particularly violent patient?
Brian Ward

A: In 1870 the treatment of psychiatric patients had progressed little since the Dark Ages in many places. In others a more compassionate approach had been adopted. Still, since psychiatric diseases were (and still are in many respects) discomforting and bizarre to most people, treatment in 1870 remained archaic by today's standards.

At that time psychiatric diseases were still seen as the result of "bad air," miasmas, spells, "uncleanliness," repayment for past sins, proof of demonic possession, or evidence that the person was a practitioner of witchcraft. Treatment consisted of incarceration and often punishment. Everything from herbs and honey to ice baths were used. Belladonna, alcohol, barbiturates, tincture of opium, and laudanum (also a form of opium) were used to sedate the crazy, angry, rowdy, and psychotic. Interestingly, some of the side effects of each of these, especially belladonna, were bizarre behavior, delusional thinking, confusion, disorientation, hallucinations, and even seizures. Each of these side effects could be viewed as further proof of an unclean or sinful existence or of demonic possession, and further punishment could then be rightly delivered.

In 1870 psychotherapy was a new concept, hypnotism was just beginning to make a stir, and Sigmund Freud, born in 1856, was only fourteen years old and still years away from his transforming theories.

As far as drug therapy for psychiatric patients, the barbiturates were available in 1870 but did not come into common use until the first half of the twentieth century. It was not until the 1950s that tranquilizers and antidepressants reached the market. Barbiturates were replaced by the class of drugs known as benzodiazepines (Valium, Xanax, etc.) in the 1960s and 1970s and this trend continues today. The first truly antipsychotic medication, Thorazine (chlorpromazine), did not appear until 1953.

The bottom line is that your character might be treated with compassion or be locked up as an animal and physically and psychologically abused. If he needed controlling it would likely be with a combination of restraints and sedation with opium or alcohol, though barbiturates might be used. If your treating physicians were on the cutting edge of current treatment, your character might receive some rudimentary psychotherapy, or might even be hypnotized.

Was Polio Present in the United States in the 1890s?

Q: For my work in progress I need to know if polio was a fairly common disease in the mid-Atlantic in the 1890–1900 era? If so, what symptoms/effects might it create in a previously healthy sixty-year-old male? Confinement to a wheelchair? Premature aging?

A: Yes, poliomyelitis was present in the United States during that time period. It was not common in 1890, but several epidemics swept through the United States during the twentieth century. The earliest was 1916 and the last was 1961. The worst was 1952, when fifty-eight thousand cases were reported.

It is a neurological disease that is caused by a virus. The initial symptoms are fever, chills, malaise, sore throat, headache, anorexia (loss of appetite), and myalgias (muscular soreness). These symptoms resolve in about three days, and the victim then feels fine. Very much like the flu, and indeed this may be the end of it. Or not.

Neurological symptoms and signs, such as a gradual weakness that may be asymmetric (one side or one leg or arm weaker than the other), may appear. This weakness tends to affect the larger muscles more than the smaller ones. This means that the thigh and shoulder muscles may be weaker than those of the forearm or lower leg. Paralysis often follows. After the large muscles begin to lose their function, the muscles involved in speech, swallowing, and breathing become weak, and ultimately lose their function. In the 1950s, "iron lungs" were used to support respiration, but in 1890 these were not available.

Polio kills by its paralysis, which also involves the muscles used for respiration. This leads to asphyxia and death. This could happen to your victim, or the process could be less severe, and he could continue to breathe, survive the acute illness, and even return to normal over time. Or he could be left with permanent paralysis of a leg or arm.

The variable ways polio affects different people gives you many options for your story. Your character could seem to have the flu and recover completely; could develop mild polio with weakness or paralysis of an arm or a leg (which could be temporary or permanent); could develop severe paralysis but be able to breathe (and suffer long-term incapacity); or he could develop severe polio and die from asphyxia due to paralysis of his breathing muscles.

How Fast Could an Aerosolized Virus Incapacitate a Person?

Q: I've finished an aviation thriller, and I have a couple of medical questions. What is the fastest-acting virus in humans in terms of time from initial infection to display of symptoms? Is it feasible for a virus, such as a filovirus, delivered by an aerosol, to debilitate a character within minutes?

> Dick Vojvoda
> Danville, California
> Author of *The Gate to Hell*

A: You are correct to consider one of the filoviruses, which are divided into two groups, Ebola and Marburg. There are subgroups of each type, and they are all very rapidly acting viruses. So far so good. But how rapid is rapid? Let's look at how viruses work.

Viruses are basically inert, meaning that by themselves they can do little. They consist of strands of DNA or RNA packaged in a protein shell. To cause problems in humans, the virus must enter the body and take up residence within the body's cells. Once inside they use the cell's own enzymes and energy-producing structures to cause an inflammatory reaction within the body. It's complicated physiology but it's this inflammation, along with the body's own immune responses to the virus, that causes most of the mischief. These inflammatory responses are the *itises* that you are familiar with. *Itis* in medicine means inflammation. So pharyngitis is an inflammation of the pharynx (throat), pleuritis is of the pleura (the lining of the lungs), gastritis is of the stomach, pericarditis is of the pericardium (the sac around the heart), meningitis is of the meninges (the membrane around the brain), and so forth.

The point is that all this inflammation takes time. The time between infection and symptoms is the incubation period, and it varies from virus to virus and from person to person. For filoviruses this incubation period is from two to twenty days.

So a virus spray might infect someone, but it would not cause any immediate reaction. A chemical such as an acid or a poison, such as cyanide, might, but not an infectious agent. Infections of all kinds take time to develop.

What Injuries from a Gunshot or a Stabbing Render a Woman Unable to Bear Children?

Q: I have two female characters in my novel, both of whom experience trauma to their abdominal region, one a gunshot, the other a stabbing. Both undergo surgery, spend time in the ICU, require colostomies for a while, and though they recover fully, no longer have the capacity to bear children. I assume they might have complete hysterectomies. If so, would the surgeon have time to harvest eggs for later use with a surrogate? Finally, what kind of physical therapy and home care would be required once they are released from the hospital? How much time would they need before returning to normal physical activities like jogging and playing softball?

A: Trauma is of two major types—blunt or penetrating. Blunt trauma is a fist to the face or a baseball bat to the head. Penetrating trauma is a bullet or knife to the belly or an arrow to the back. Your victims suffer penetrating trauma. The nature of the exact injuries depends upon what internal organs are involved.

Rapid death would occur only if a major blood vessel such as the aorta or vena cava within the abdomen were damaged. Otherwise the victim would survive and would be treated surgically to control bleeding and to repair any damaged organs. The liver, stomach, pancreas, and spleen lie in the upper part of the abdomen, while the intestines, kidneys, and bladder lie in the middle and lower portions. Which of these organs are injured would depend upon where the bullet or blade entered the belly and how deeply it penetrated. The resulting surgery would likewise depend upon what structures were injured.

If the colon or intestines were injured, the surgical repair might include resection (removal) of a portion of the bowel and a reanastomosis (rejoining) of the two parts. A colostomy is the redirecting of the bowel from its normal attachment to the anus through the abdominal wall. A colostomy bag is placed over the opening to collect the stool. This procedure may or may not be necessary, depending upon the exact location and severity of the bowel injury. When done a colostomy may be temporary—a few weeks or months—or permanent. Your two ladies could easily require a temporary colostomy.

If the uterus were injured so severely that it could not be repaired, a hysterectomy might be necessary. In such a medical emergency, egg harvesting would not take place. Besides, egg harvesting requires weeks or months of preparation with hormones to stimulate the production of many eggs for the harvesting procedure. These hormones and drugs are what are commonly called "fertility drugs." In the circumstance where the uterus is injured and a hysterectomy is performed, the ovaries would most likely be left in place. So even though they could not become pregnant, either of your characters could later undergo this preparation, and the eggs could be harvested using a laparoscope. Then the eggs could be fertilized and a surrogate mother could carry the fetus. So biological motherhood is still possible, just not in the usual way.

The length of recovery would depend upon the victim's age and general health, the nature of the injuries, and the extent of the surgery required to repair the injuries. In general, a couple of days in the ICU, followed by three to six more days in the hospital, followed by two to six weeks of recovery would be likely. Physical therapy would consist mostly of help with walking and daily care issues, such as bathing, dressing, and feeding. This may be for a few days or several weeks, again depending upon the nature and extent of the injuries and surgery.

If all went well the victims could return to normal activities in two to four weeks, and to some low level of exercise in six to eight weeks. It may take three or four months for full recovery. These are general time estimates, and highly variable.

Was the Technology Available in the 1980s to Keep a Pregnant Woman in a Vegetative State Alive Long Enough to Deliver Her Child?

Q: My story takes place twenty to twenty-five years ago. If a pregnant woman is critically injured in an accident and left in a permanent, vegetative state, could she be kept alive for the baby's sake?

Lee Goldberg

Los Angeles, California

Author of the Diagnosis Murder and Monk series

www.leegoldberg.com

A: Yes. Some people in this state, like the late Terri Schiavo in Florida, are not on any life support such as ventilators. These individuals only require food, water, and basic care. They can live for decades this way. Death is usually from infections, with urinary tract infections and pneumonias being the most common. Even if your victim were on a ventilator, the care would be the same, except that ventilator management comes into play and the risk of pneumonia is increased. With proper care and good luck people can live a long time in this situation.

What you describe has happened more than once. It is a "right-to-life" issue for many, so it is now wrapped in politics, but medically a woman can be kept alive until the child is ready for delivery. This means the child should be twenty-eight or more weeks old. The longer the physicians can delay, the more mature the child will be, and the better chance it has of survival. Let's say your woman is seven months along. Keep her alive for another month or six weeks, do a C-section to remove the baby, and then a decision can be made about whether to remove the mother's life support or not.

Twenty-five years ago the technology needed to do this was available.

How Would a Bear Bite Be Treated in a Wilderness Area?

Q: I have a healthy male character traveling in a mountainous area in 1880. He is mauled by a grizzly bear in the shoulder. I want there to be lots of bleeding. Can he be nicked in an artery where he needs more than just pressure to stop the flow, or will that nick kill him? I was thinking that his companion might heat a knife blade and use the heated steel to "seal" the wound. Would that work, or is this an unrealistic situation?

Cat Dubie
Surrey, British Columbia, Canada

A: This works very well. There are several arteries in the shoulder, some are large, others smaller. He could easily have one of the smaller arteries damaged and bleed significantly. His companion could first apply pressure but see that the bleeding is continuing despite this. He could then use the heated knife to cauterize (burn) the wound. This would seal the vessel and stop the bleeding. The major threat to his health would then be an infection in the wound. This may or may not happen, so you can have it either way in your story. If you want him to live, no infection; if you want him to die, have an infection set in.

Can an Overly Aggressive Chiropractic Adjustment Lead to Death?

Q: I am working on a short story in which a part-time instructor at a college has given up waiting for a position to open and has decided to eliminate a few full-timers. His first victim goes to a chiropractor on a regular basis. The protagonist slips in, dresses in a doctor's tunic, pretends to do a neck adjustment, and breaks the victim's neck. Could this work? Would the autopsy show that it was a murder instead of a "treatment"?

Don Moore
Santa Clarita, California

A: Any twisting force to the neck that is powerful enough can fracture one or more of the cervical vertebrae (neck spinal bones). And any fracture of these bones can damage the spinal cord and lead to paralysis or death. And though it's not common, it can and does happen with chiropractic manipulations.

If the cord were transected (cut in half) by the fractured bones, the victim would immediately lose consciousness and fall into what we call spinal shock. In this situation the blood pressure immediately and severely plummets, breathing ceases, and the victim dies from asphyxia and shock. If the cord is merely bruised or slightly torn, the victim may survive but suffer partial paralysis, weakness of one side of the body or one limb, numbness of one side or one limb, and many other symptoms. These may be permanent, or may partially or completely resolve over a few days, weeks, or months. Almost anything can happen and over almost any time frame, so you have a lot to work with if you decide to go this route, as opposed to death of the victim.

At autopsy the ME could determine that the vertebrae were fractured, that the spinal cord was injured, and that this was the cause of death. What he could not determine is who did it and why. Was it accidental or homicidal? That's what the police would investigate and the court would decide.

What Early-1900s Folk Remedies Were Effective for Controlling Bleeding?

Q: In my 1930s story a mother must stop the bleeding from a minor cut on her five-year-old daughter's arm. What herb or other folk remedy might she have used?

A: There are several that may or may not be truly effective but have been used over the years. Obviously, these would have a chance of working only in cases of minor bleeding. Severe bleeding is another situation entirely.

> **Eggs:** Egg white was often smeared on wounds. Sometimes the whites would be mixed with honey or flour or sugar. The proteins in the egg white may have some coagulant properties. Also, the thin membrane that lines the inside of the eggshell can be carefully peeled away and placed over the wound. In addition to supplying a coagulating protein, this may also work as a "seal" to help arrest blood flow. My mother would use this technique on boils and bee stings, too.

> **Mud:** A thick mud was used to stop bleeding many years ago, before the germ theory became part of our knowledge base. It works as a barrier, slowing blood flow and allowing the body's natural clotting mechanism to take over. Secondary infection is a problem here. This was still used in the 1930s.

> **Tobacco:** A mixture of tobacco and water (or spit) can be applied like a paste. Again, there is a barrier effect. Also, tobacco would make a good antiseptic and would kill many common bacteria in this concentrated form. Perhaps more important, nicotine is a vasoconstrictor (narrows the blood vessels) and would thus reduce blood flow and help with clot formation.

> **Herbs:** Just about any plant material you can think of has been used. The sap of the aloe plant is still a component

of many burn and bruise treatments. Also, the flowers and roots of the *Arnica montana* (Wolfsbane, Leopards-bane, mountain tobacco) plant have been touted as having the capacity to stop bleeding and aid with wound healing. It grows in Europe, particularly the Alps of Switzerland, and in the mountains of Canada and the northern portions of the United States. A mixture of crushed leaves or roots with water would be applied to the wound.

Your mother could use any or all of these home remedies.

Was Toxemia a Recognized Medical Condition in the 1890s?

Q: I'm writing a novel set in the American Midwest in the late nineteenth century. I plan to have one of my characters develop toxemia during pregnancy and die because of it. But was pregnancy-related toxemia a recognized condition in the 1890s? Did doctors have an understanding of high blood pressure and its effects back then? Also, was what we now call "asthma" known by that name in the last quarter of the nineteenth century?

A: Yes. Both toxemia and puerperal sepsis (uterine and blood infection that occurs around the time of delivery and after) were both known problems of pregnancy. And neither had effective treatment at that time and caused many peri-partum (around the time of delivery) deaths. The woman with toxemia (now called eclampsia and preeclampsia, depending on the severity) would develop high blood pressure, edema (ankle swelling), headaches, irritability, photophobia (light hurts the eyes), nervousness, anxiety, and if severe, seizures, coma, and death.

Your young lady could develop any or all of these symptoms, and the local doctor could do little about them. Maybe he would recommend laudanum (tincture of opium) for pain and sedation, or he might even perform bloodletting, which actually might be of some benefit. For a while anyway. The family would likely try various herbs and elixirs, and probably resort to prayer. But the process would continue, and your young lady would ultimately suffer seizures, coma, and death—unless she went into labor and delivered or aborted the child. This would "cure" the eclampsia, and she would likely do well if she survived what would be a very rocky childbirth or miscarriage.

Blood pressure was first measured by Stephen Hales in 1733, and was first recorded on a kymograph in 1847 by Carl Ludwig. The measuring devices available then were very bulky, and it wasn't until 1881 that Samuel Siegfried Karl von Basch invented the sphygmomanometer, the precursor of the modern blood pressure cuff. It was years before these reached wide use, so it is very unlikely that one of these devices would be available to a physician in your story. And even though the blood pressure was measurable in 1890, little was known about how detrimental hypertension truly was, and no treatment was available.

Asthma has been known for centuries if not millennia. Again, in the 1890s there was no treatment, and deaths were not rare.

Why Did Physicians Begin to Wash Their Hands Before Delivering Babies?

Q: I am in the process of finishing a nonfiction book and have been pursuing Ignaz Semmelweis's work regarding washing hands prior to delivering babies to reduce infection, disease, and death. I read that he had a name for this that was something equivalent to "just because you cannot 'see it' doesn't mean that it is not there." Any help you can give me in this regard is greatly appreciated.

A: The infectious process you are referring to is called puerperal sepsis. This is a uterine infection following childbirth. It is due to bacteria entering the uterus during the delivery process.

During the early 1800s the germ theory for infections had not been established, and many theories existed to explain how infections occurred and were spread. One was the theory of miasmas, which were "evil vapors" that were thought to carry disease into the human. They were actually evil only in that prayer was believed to be more important to avoiding them than any known medical intervention. Then Antoni van Leeuwenhoek (1632–1723) invented the microscope and saw what he called "little animals." These were actually bacteria. He had no idea what, if anything, they did.

Ignaz Philipp Semmelweis (1818–1865) noticed that women who were delivered by midwives suffered fewer postpartum infections than did those delivered by physicians or medical students. He further noted that midwives washed their hands more frequently, and in general adhered more closely to the principles of general cleanliness. After instituting simple hand washing before delivery, the incidence of infection dropped dramatically. Semmelweis still possessed no concept of bacteria as the cause of disease but had made the empiric observation that hand washing lessened infections in this situation.

The theory to which you are referring may be spontaneous generation, which means that bacteria arose from nothing. That is, they spontaneously appeared within wounds. This theory held sway for some time and had to be disproved before the germ theory could take over. The work of people such as Robert Koch, Louis Pasteur, and Joseph Lister was developed into the germ theory of disease as we now know it.

How Would a Smallpox Outbreak on a Sailing Ship Psychologically Impact the Crew?

Q: I am working on a nonfiction book for middle-school readers that deals with daily life on voyages to the New World in the sixteenth and seventeenth centuries. I'm familiar with how smallpox spreads and its symptoms, but I'm wondering about its emotional impact on the crew. Most diarists of the time are rather unemotional.

Any idea how an outbreak might affect the crew?

Andrew A. Kling

Great Falls, Montana

Author of *Life on a New World Voyage*

A: Smallpox is a serious disease that carries a 30 to 40 percent mortality rate even with good care, and it would have been much higher in the time period of your research. It tends to occur in epidemics that strike an area quickly and hard. The victims develop a blistery rash that is very disfiguring in the survivors. Those who die often develop pneumonia, and this is what ultimately does them in. It commonly decimated crews, at times killing well over half of the sailors.

During the sixteenth and seventeenth centuries absolutely nothing was known about the cause, manner of contagion and spread, or treatment of smallpox. The germ theory was still centuries away. Instead, this deadly and disfiguring disease, and most other diseases, were believed to be the work of God, the devil, evil spirits, bad air, miasmas, poisons, impure thoughts, hexes and spells, witches' brews, you name it. Thus victims were treated as unclean, impure, evil, and un-Godly. They were avoided, tossed from society, and even killed.

In a closed environment such as a ship at sea, panic and terror would be the rule of the day. Victims could be merely quarantined, or tossed overboard. They could be tortured or exorcised. The ship would likely become a house divided, with mutiny and warfare among the crew. Only two basic things motivate people: need and fear. By far fear is more powerful, and drives people to do awful things. And fear would be rampant on the ship.

What Happens When Someone Is Exposed to the Vacuum of Space?

Q: What sort of damage does the human body suffer in the vacuum of space? How long can one survive, and what will happen to the person who does survive? My

scenario involves an astronaut whose faceplate blows
out, but not before he depressurizes his suit sufficiently
to prevent immediate death.

Justin L. Peniston
Los Angeles, California
www.quixoticcomics.com

A: First of all, the victim would not explode as is the case in
many movies. But some really bad things do happen internally, and
they happen very quickly. Whether he depressurizes somewhat
beforehand or not, his survival would likely be measured in seconds, a minute or two at the outside.

Space decompression is similar to that of a scuba diver who rises
too rapidly after a prolonged exposure to the pressures of the deep.
In this case he is going from excess pressure to normal pressure. In
space the victim goes from normal pressure to zero pressure. Same
thing physiologically.

Though studies on the effects of exposure to a vacuum have
been done on chimpanzees, there are no real data on what happens
to humans exposed to zero pressure except for a couple of incidents where an astronaut or a pilot was accidentally exposed. Of
course, rapid decompression has caused deaths in both high-
altitude flights and, in June 1971, when the Russian spacecraft
Soyuz 11 suddenly lost pressure and killed the three cosmonauts
onboard.

On August 16, 1960, parachutist Joe Kittinger ascended to an
altitude of 102,800 feet (19.5 miles) in an open gondola in order to
set a world record for high-altitude parachute jumping. He lost
pressurization in his right glove but proceeded with his ascent and
jump. He experienced pain and loss of function in his hand at high
altitude, but all returned to normal once he descended via chute to
lower altitudes.

In 1965 at NASA's Manned Spacecraft Center near Houston,
Texas, a trainee suffered a sudden leak in his space suit while in a
vacuum chamber. He lost consciousness in fourteen seconds, but
revived after a few seconds as the chamber was immediately repres-
surized. He suffered no ill effects from his very brief exposure, but

stated that he could feel water boiling on his tongue. I should point out that in chemical and physical terms boiling simply means the changing of a liquid to a gas. This can be accomplished by adding heat or by lowering the ambient air pressure. So in this case it wasn't that his tongue became hot but rather that the pressure was so low the water in his mouth changed to its gaseous phase.

A case of partial, prolonged exposure occurred during an EVA (extravehicular activity, or space walk) in April 1991 on the U.S. space shuttle mission STS-37. One astronaut suffered a ⅛-inch puncture in one glove between the thumb and forefinger. He was unaware of it until later, when he noticed a painful red mark on his skin in the exposed area. It appeared that the area had bled some but that his blood had clotted and sealed the injury.

So, what happens to a human exposed to zero pressure? Since there is no oxygen in such an environment, loss of consciousness occurs in a matter of seconds. Also, if the victim held his breath (don't do this during scuba diving when coming up from depths either), the air in his lungs would rapidly expand and his lungs could be damaged, bleed, or rupture. Better to open his mouth and exhale the rapidly expanding gas from the lungs.

Water in his bloodstream would immediately begin to boil. That is, it would turn into its gaseous state. This is similar to popping the top on a soft drink. With the release of the pressure the carbon dioxide dissolved in the drink immediately begins to turn into its gas form. Same thing happens in the blood at zero pressure. This causes pressure to build in the blood system, and the heart stops. Bubbles may appear in the bloodstream, and these can cause damage to the body's organs, particularly the brain. As a result, the brain and nerves cease to function. This increased pressure also causes the tissues of the body to swell, maybe even to split or tear, but they will not explode.

But what if the exposure is brief and the person is rescued? Treatment would be to immediately return him to a pressurized environment and give him 100 percent oxygen. He may survive unharmed, or may have brain and nerve damage, which could be permanent.

For your scenario the victim's faceplate would rupture, and he would begin to exhale air. He would lose consciousness in ten to twenty seconds, and would then die in short order. If he were rescued quickly, he would be returned to the spacecraft, which would be pressurized, and he would be given 100 percent oxygen via a face mask. He could survive intact or with brain damage. It's your call. Either way works.

Part II

Poisons, Toxins, Medications, and Drugs

Is There a Drug That Would Cause Amnesia?

Q: My antagonist wants to induce temporary amnesia in my heroine by giving her a drug. Is there a chemical that could cause the amnesia yet allow for some recovery of memory shortly after discontinuing it? I need the drug to be given in food or drink, cause little sedation, have few side effects, and make it possible for him to "reprogram" her into being someone else. Am I way off base here?

A: There is no drug that exactly fits your needs, but there are several that will work. All the sedatives and narcotics that might cause amnesia (morphine, heroin, Valium, and others) would make the victim very sleepy and lethargic, so they won't work for you. A drug used as a preanesthetic agent called Versed could work. It does not make the victim sleepy, but it would essentially erase any memory of events that occur while she's under its influence. But it must be injected, either intramuscularly (IM) or intravenously (IV), so this doesn't fit your needs either.

However, the category of chemicals known as date rape drugs fit your scenario. Each of these can prevent memory and may or may not cause any noticeable sedation. For example, Ecstasy may cause the victim to become talkative and happy but not necessarily "drunk." Or it may cause extreme sedation, loss of coordination, and coma. It's unpredictable, which means you can have it either way in your story.

Small amounts added to food or drink over a period of time would definitely scramble the victim's perceptions of ongoing events and memories of events that occurred while under the influence of the drug. Afterward, portions of the victim's memory could spontaneously come back slowly, or not at all. It could return in fits and spurts, or very suddenly as a result of some trigger. Hypnosis might help recover some memories. This gives you several ways to retrieve the information your character needs.

Any of the date rape drugs can cause sedation, confusion, euphoria, loss of identity, dizziness, blurred vision, slowed movements and reflexes, and amnesia. The victim often will have poor judgment and become highly suggestible. This means that your villain could talk her into almost anything. For your purposes the most important effects of these drugs is amnesia.

The most common date rape drugs are:

> **Rohypnol** (street names: roofies, roaches, rope, Mexican Valium): a benzodiazepine sedative in the same family as Valium, was developed to treat insomnia. Currently the drug is neither manufactured nor approved for use in the United States, but is available in Mexico and many other countries. It is manufactured as white, one- and two-milligram tablets that can be crushed and dissolved in any liquid. It takes action twenty to thirty minutes after ingestion, peaks in about two hours, and its effects may persist for eight to twelve hours.

> **Ecstasy** (street names: E, X, XTC, MDMA, love, Adam): originally patented in 1914 as an appetite suppressant; was never marketed. It is currently manufactured in underground labs and distributed in pill or capsule form. It has amphetamine (speedlike) as well as hallucinogenic effects. Rare cases of death from malignant hyperthermia (sudden and marked elevation of body temperature to 106–108 degrees, or above, which basically "fries" the brain) have been reported.

> **GHB** (street names: G, XTC, E, liquid ecstasy, liquid E, easy lay, goop, scoop, Georgia Home Boy): developed over thirty years ago; was sold as a "natural" food supplement and muscle builder. It comes as a white powder that dis-

solves easily in water, alcohol, and other liquids. It is also available as "liquid E," a colorless, odorless liquid that is sold in small vials and bottles. The effects of GHB appear five to twenty minutes after ingestion and typically last for two to three hours.

One of the problems users face is that both Ecstasy and GHB are often called Ecstasy, though they are very different compounds. The street purchaser doesn't always know which he is getting. Both are often cooked up in a garage by someone of unknown expertise, marginal experience, questionable drug habits, and with an outdated chemistry book.

Ketamine (street names: K, special K, kit-kat, purple, bump): a rapid-acting IV or IM surgical anesthetic agent commonly used in the 1970s. It fell from favor in part due to its unpredictable hallucinogenic and psychiatric side effects. It is still occasionally used medically in burn victims since it tends to dissociate the patient from the pain, making the intense discomfort of burns more bearable. It is popular in veterinary clinics as an animal sedative, leading to another popular street name, Cat Valium. In fact, the Ketamine that appears on the street is often stolen from animal hospitals and clinics.

Ketamine comes as a liquid, which can be heated and evaporated, leaving a white powder residue. The powder can be added to a liquid such as a bottle of water, compacted into pills, or snorted, which is the preferred and most common method of usage. When snorted it takes effect almost immediately and is fairly short in its duration of action, forty-five minutes to an hour or two.

In Ketamine's dissociative effects the user experiences hallucinations, loss of time sense, and loss of self-identity. One common form is a depersonalization syndrome where the person is part of the activities while at the same time is off to the side or hovering overhead watching the activity, including his/her own actions. This reaction is also common with PCP (phencyclidine, or angel dust). Users call these effects "going into a K Hole."

Any of these should work for you but Ecstasy, Rohypnol, and GHB would be your best bets. Your victim would appear normal, or perhaps slightly intoxicated or sleepy, and would have little or no memory of what happened. Her memory may be recoverable or not, depending on what you need for your story.

Can a Single Drink of Alcohol Harm or Kill a Nondrinker?

Q: I am writing a short story in which a professional football player is given something in his drink that sends him away from a party feeling sick or drunk. He is against drug use of any kind, including caffeine. I'm not sure yet if it's the drink and its substance that kills him, or someone who follows him and then does him in. Could enough alcohol in a single drink make him severely disoriented? Kill him? Could he be allergic to the alcohol? If he dies from either the alcohol or an attack would alcohol show up in his blood?

Judy Clemens
Anthony- and Agatha-award-nominated author of the
   Stella Crown series
www.judyclemens.com

A: It would be virtually impossible for a single drink, even if it was pure, 200-proof grain alcohol, to kill someone, and alcohol allergies are very rare. A single drink might make a nondrinker tipsy, even goofy, but would not kill him. It could interfere with his judgment, which could cause him to wander into a dangerous situation, where he could be killed or harmed.

I would suggest adding something to the alcoholic drink. In fact, the drink wouldn't even have to contain alcohol. The date rape drugs Ecstasy, GHB, Rohypnol, and Ketamine would all work.

They are available on the street and can easily be slipped into a drink. They have no taste, so the drinker would not know. And it only takes a small amount. Any of these could cause the person to appear inebriated and cloud his judgment, even more than a couple of drinks of alcohol would. And a very large dose of any of them could be deadly. The main effect of these drugs is that they make the person highly suggestible. Your victim could easily be lead or tricked into a situation where he could be killed or harmed. And if he survived an assault, his memory would be absent or spotty.

Alcohol is very easily detected in the blood at almost any level in both the living and the dead. And if you added one of the above drugs, they would also be detected by toxicological examination.

Can the Type of Alcohol a Victim Has Consumed Be Determined at Autopsy?

Q: I am working on a story in which someone drowns while very intoxicated. Can a medical examiner determine how much and what kind of alcohol is present in a victim's blood? If the corpse is not found for eight hours will there still be alcohol in his blood, or does it break down?

Paul Yeuell

Hollywood, California

Television writing staff, researcher, CBS's *Cold Case*

A: The short answer is, most likely.

If the victim had taken enough alcohol to cause intoxication, his tissues and stomach contents would reflect this. Since all metabolism (the breakdown of toxins and foods) ceases at death, the alcohol would not undergo any conversion by the body itself. At least, not enough for its level to decline appreciably. Toxicological testing for alcohol is done easily and is highly accurate, so the ME could determine the exact level of the alcohol within the victim. In suspected alcohol-caused deaths, or in deaths where alcohol intoxication might be a factor, the ME can measure the alcohol level in the cadaver's blood and urine (typically blood is used and is the most accurate determinant) and tell if the intoxication level was high enough to have caused or contributed to the death. In your scenario if he found a very high level of alcohol he might conclude that the intoxication was an important factor in the drowning. If he found a low level he might conclude the opposite—that alcohol had little or nothing to do with the drowning.

There are, however, a few situations where this testing may be inaccurate. If the body undergoes putrefaction (decay due to bacteria), and if this process is so far along (days or weeks, not eight hours) that the tissues are severely broken down, then the alcohol may also be consumed in this decay process to a degree that the ME can't be sure what the premortem level actually was. And with severe decay the alcohol level may actually *increase* due to the action of the putrefying bacteria, some of which produce alcohol as a by-product of their activity. Go figure.

To get around this, a determination of the alcohol level in the vitreous fluid of the eye would be done. This is the fluid within the eyeball, and it is called the vitreous humor—not as in funny but as in the old humors of Aristotle. Some things in medicine never die. The alcohol level in the vitreous humor reflects the blood alcohol level with a one- to two-hour lag. That is, it can tell the ME what the blood level was one to two hours before death, but not right at death. This allows him to make a "best guess" as to the level of intoxication at the time of death, and since this is all ballpark anyway, this estimation usually suffices.

In your scenario the ME would have a fairly intact corpse, since little decay would occur in only eight hours. He would test the blood, urine, stomach contents, and possibly the vitreous fluid, and uncover the type and amount of alcohol present.

Regarding the type of alcohol, he could determine that the alcohol was ethanol (drinking alcohol) as opposed to methanol (wood or denatured alcohol) or isopropanol (rubbing alcohol). But using blood, urine, or vitreous fluid, he could not tell what type of drinking alcohol was consumed. Ethanol is ethanol. Beer, wine, and whiskey all contain the same alcohol and all look the same in the blood. But if the stomach contents are analyzed it is at least possible that he could distinguish beer from wine from vodka. Not from the alcohol in these beverages but from the other chemicals that make wine wine and beer beer. Or he may not be able to determine this. It can go either way.

Would an Injected Anticoagulant Make Someone Bleed More Severely from Knife Wounds?

Q: My killer hangs his victim by the heels over a tub, injects him with an anticoagulant, and then inflicts a series of knife wounds so that the victim bleeds to death. The room is very warm and the corpse is not found for a couple of days. Would the blood in the tub be congealed by then? Will it ever congeal, or will it stay "thinned"? What might it look like?

> Jan Burke
> Edgar Award–winning author of *Nine* and *Bloodlines*
> www.janburke.com

A: The injectable anticoagulant you need is called heparin and is used widely in hospitals. It could be stolen easily from a hospital pharmacy or medical ward, or it could be purchased through a pharmacy or pharmaceutical supply house. It is not a controlled substance, so it is readily available.

It works immediately after injection intravenously (IV). In your scenario I would have the villain give the victim 100,000 units IV, then do his dirty deeds. The victim would bleed profusely from almost any wound and would exsanguinate (bleed to death) fairly quickly.

The blood would never clot, and would remain liquid for the two days, but would of course begin to putrefy just as the body would. After two days in a very warm environment the blood would be liquid, reddish-brown, and might show significant bacterial growth, which might make it cloudy. It and the body would possess a putrid odor.

The ME should be able to determine that heparin was present if he thought to test for it. If the blood and the corpse were fresh, the fact that the blood was still unclotted might push him to search out why, and he would uncover the heparin. But if both the blood and the corpse were severely decayed, as in your very warm room scenario, he might not, and simply write off the liquid nature of the blood to the decay process.

What Toxin Can Be Administered Over Time and Cause Death with Symptoms That Would Mimic a Stroke?

Q: I am writing a murder mystery where a man is fed a poison for a month or two that would cause strokelike symptoms such as impaired speech and weakness. It also has to be metabolized by the body so that it does not leave traces, as arsenic does. The death takes place in New Orleans, so I was hoping to find some kind of native plant.

Wendy Nelson (writing as Lawana Edwards)
Shakopee, Minnesota

A: Most killers who use poisons prefer fast-acting ones. This is to make sure it works, and because they may not have repeated or prolonged access to the victim. Family members, roommates, and others close to the victim do have long-term access, so chronic poisoning does occur. Your scenario requires a chronic poison that has neurological effects.

There are several possibilities for your scenario, but the most common and readily available are what we call heavy metals. These are things such as arsenic (AS), mercury (Hg), and lead (Pb). I know you did not want to use AS, but it's common because it works, and is often overlooked as the cause of death. Basically you want a drug or chemical that causes a slow death with neurological features and is not readily detected. Let's look at why the heavy metals might work for your story.

The chronic ingestion of any of these heavy metals would cause the gradual onset of symptoms such as fatigue, nausea, vomiting, diarrhea (bloody or not), weight loss, shortness of breath, headaches, numbness, weakness of the muscles, confusion, and disorientation. Strength, balance, walking ability, and speech can be affected, and these symptoms can mimic neurological problems, including strokes. The victim's M.D. would not think of metal poisoning at first, and maybe not at all. He would evaluate the victim for ulcers, gastroenteritis, colitis (an inflammation of the colon), neurological diseases, strokes, kidney infection, cancer of the stomach or colon, viruses (including AIDS), and other disorders. The workup would all be normal, and he might assume the victim had a prolonged viral illness.

Yes, each of these metals is easily found in the body of a victim, but even with modern forensic techniques people often get away with poisoning, because it is not thought of. If an eighty-five-year-old demented person with heart and lung disease dies in his sleep in a nursing home, the person's private M.D. would sign the death certificate as a natural cardiac death, and the ME would accept it. Likely no autopsy would be done, and no toxicological exams would be undertaken. An overdose of morphine or digitalis, the actual cause of death, would go undetected. But if a five-million-dollar inheritance were in play, and if the insurance company didn't have to pay for a victim of murder, or if one family member suspected another, the ME might be asked to open a file and investigate.

So the first step in your killer getting away with a poisoning murder is to make it look like something else. Keep the ME completely out of the picture, or at least give him an easy answer for the cause of death. If no murder is suspected he'll take the path of least resistance, which is also the cheapest route. And he must live with and justify his budget annually. If he is wasteful he'll be looking for a job. Give him a cheap and easy out.

The second step is to use a poison that is not readily detectable by most drug screens. The heavy metals fit this scenario. Drug screens on both the living and the dead typically test for alcohol, narcotics, sedatives, marijuana, cocaine, amphetamines, and aspirin. Some screen for a few other classes. Once a member of a class is identified, further testing will be done to determine exactly which member of the class is present and in what amount. For example, if an amphetamine or narcotic is found, further testing will be done to discover exactly which amphetamine or narcotic is present. If the screen shows nothing, further testing is unlikely unless the ME is given a compelling reason to look further.

Remember that specialized toxicological tests are expensive and time consuming, and are used only if the general screen shows something. If not, the ME saves money, the death is attributed to something else, and life goes on. But if a poison is suspected, and if the funds and interest to pursue it are present, anything can be found in an intact corpse. Using gas chromatography in conjunction with either mass spectrometry (GC/MS) or infrared spectrometry (GC/IR) would give a chemical fingerprint for any molecule. And since each molecule has its own structure, and thus its own fingerprint, every compound can be distinguished from every other one.

One other point to consider is that these metals can be detected in the victim's hair if it is tested. And this testing would give a timeline for the exposure. Let me explain. Only the hair produced at the time the blood level of the metal was high would contain the metal. So if the poisoning was intermittent and the victim's hair was analyzed, the level found in the hair would vary along its length. Segments formed when the level of the metal was high in the blood would show higher levels, while those formed when the level was low would reveal lower levels. This way a timeline of exposure can be determined.

So you can have your villain use one of the heavy metals, disguise the death as something else, and she just might get away with it. Until your sleuth figures out something is amiss and nudges the ME to dig a little deeper.

Another possibility for your scenario is either the English yew (*Taxus baccata*) or the Japanese yew (*Taxus cuspidate*). Both are very toxic plants. The toxin in both is taxine, a mixture of alkaloids. It causes neurological (numbness, weakness, loss of balance, etc.) and cardiac problems, and typically kills by causing a cardiac arrest.

Taxol (paclitaxel) is manufactured by Bristol-Myers Squibb and comes in vials of 6 mgs/ml. It is a semisynthetic drug made from *Taxus baccata,* and thus its toxic effects are similar to those of taxine, and it kills in the same fashion. It is used in the treatment of breast cancer, so your villain could get access to such a drug if this is a plot element. It can be detected in the victim's blood and tissues, but again, only if the ME looks for it.

Saxitoxin would also work for you. It is classified as a PSP, or paralytic shellfish poison, is produced by certain algae, and is the toxin involved in red tide intoxications. It is similar to other marine toxins, such as those of the blue-ringed octopus and the puffer fish (tetrodotoxin), and is very toxic, estimated to be a thousand times more toxic than the treacherous sarin, a chemical weapon terrorists used in the Tokyo subway attack.

The toxin is produced by bacteria that grow on other organisms, such as the phytoplankton algal species known as dinoflagellates *Gonyaulax catenella* and *G. tamarensis*. These algae are in turn consumed by the Alaskan butter clam and the California sea mussel. When these shellfish are ingested by humans, intoxication occurs. The toxin can be isolated from these shellfish species as well as be artificially synthesized.

Saxitoxin is used in nerve conduction studies, and in the 1950s the CIA began experimenting with its effects. During the cold war it apparently was carried in capsule form by U2 pilots such as Francis Gary Powers as a means of suicide if captured.

As a neurotoxin Saxitoxin attacks the nervous system. Its onset of action is within ten minutes, but could take up to an hour if ingested, or sooner if inhaled. There are no reported cases in the medical literature of human inhalation, but animal studies have revealed that death after inhalation occurs within a few minutes. By two hours after ingestion the symptoms are pronounced, and death can occur in two to twelve hours if the dose is sufficient, and if the victim is not treated appropriately.

Saxitoxin blocks nerve transmission at the neuromuscular junction (where the nerves attach to the muscles). Early symptoms would be giddiness, dizziness, and tingling (paresthesias) of the extremities, face, lips, and tongue. There may be mild nausea, but this is usually not prominent. These symptoms would progress to include an unstable gait, numbness and weakness of the arms and legs, slurred speech, and shortness of breath. Death can occur from cardiac arrhythmias or from respiratory paralysis.

If your perpetrator gave the victim small doses over a period of time, the victim would exhibit various neurological signs and symptoms, and would ultimately die from the toxin. And as with the others I mentioned, the ME would only find the toxin in the victim's tissues, stomach, and/or urine if he specifically looked for it. He probably wouldn't.

Is There a Drug That Paralyzes yet Leaves the Victim Fully Awake?

Q: In my story a character uses a drug that paralyzes people yet leaves them completely conscious and alert. They are unable to move or speak or scream while terrible things are done to them. Is there such a drug? If so, what's it called, and what would it be used for medically? Would there have been a variation of it available forty years ago? Would the ME be able to detect traces of it in the exhumed bodies of people who were buried forty years ago?

Lee Goldberg
Los Angeles, California
Author of the Diagnosis Murder and Monk series
www.leegoldberg.com

A: These drugs are classified as neuromuscular paralytics. They must be given by intravenous (IV) or intramuscular (IM) injection, act almost immediately, and work on the nerves or in the area where the nerves stimulate the muscles. The net effect of these drugs is that they paralyze all the muscles in the body, including those used to breathe. They do not act like sedatives or narcotics, such as morphine, alcohol, or Valium, so the victim is wide awake but literally cannot move a muscle. They can't move, speak, blink their eyes, or breathe, and die from asphyxia.

These drugs are used as part of general anesthesia. They relax the muscles so the anesthesiologist can more easily pass the endotracheal (ET) tube into the trachea and take over control of the patient's breathing. They are also used in patients with status epilepticus (uncontrolled seizure activity, which interferes with breathing). Paralyzing the person and placing them on a ventilator until the seizures can be controlled is often life saving in these cases.

There are several drugs that fit this need today, but there were two back in 1963—curare and succinylcholine (called sux for short). Sux is still commonly used today. In the past it was considered the perfect murder weapon, since it is destroyed rapidly by the body after injection, making it untraceable. Now we can measure the breakdown products of sux and prove that it was present. It has been involved in several famous cases, including the Carl Coppolino case, one of F. Lee Bailey's early legal battles. His first murder took place in 1965, using sux. It was this case that finally proved legally that sux could be identified in a corpse. Another famous case is that of Genene Jones, the Texas nurse who in the late 1970s and early 1980s gave children sux so she could then be a hero when she saved them. It took a long time to prove she was giving sux to make the kids stop breathing.

Since these drugs make the victim stop breathing, your villain should be prepared to breathe for them. He would need a ventilator to pull this off. It is sophisticated and cumbersome, so you probably want to avoid this. But a small dose of sux might make the victim so weak that movement is very difficult or impossible, but not so weak that he couldn't continue to breathe shallow breaths and remain alive. The dose to do this would be guesswork and couldn't be calculated with any accuracy, so your villain would simply give a little and see what happens.

Could the ME find the breakdown products of sux or curare in a many-decades-old corpse? Not likely, since the body would be severely decayed, if not simply a skeleton. However, if the body were very well preserved, which is possible, then maybe. The ME could take muscle, brain, and liver tissue, and if he found the injection site he could take tissue from around there (often residue of an injected drug is found around the injection site), and could test them for residual sux and for breakdown products.

Another possibility would be tetrodotoxin. This comes from the puffer fish and is used to make zombie powder, which is used in some voodoo rituals. It too has neuromuscular effects that could render the victim unable to move. His breathing would be shallow but present, unless the dose was very high. If so, the victim could die from asphyxia.

How Much Aspirin, Taken Over Several Days, Would Cause Significant Side Effects?

Q: It's 1911, London, and my fifty-seven-year-old detective has recently been diagnosed with rheumatism. At the same time a member of the royal family is kidnapped, and my detective is called upon to assist Scotland Yard in finding the missing boy. In order to keep going my detective takes too much aspirin. My questions are: How much aspirin, taken over four to five days, would cause dizziness, confusion, ringing in the ears, nausea, and vomiting without killing the detective? Would it be possible that he might become so incapacitated that his physician partner might fear for the detective's life? If so, how long would it take the iron-willed detective to recover enough to get back on the case?

John Mullen
Poway, California

A: The symptoms you describe are indeed symptoms of aspirin (acetylsalicylic acid, or ASA) toxicity. The amount required to become toxic varies widely from person to person and depends upon such things as age, size, what illnesses the person may have, what other medications he may be taking, how he reacts to and metabolizes (breaks down or destroys) medications in general and aspirin in particular, and other factors. This means that the exact amount that a particular individual must take to be harmed can't be determined accurately. The range is broad. This is good, since it allows you to construct your plot using a wide range of aspirin doses and it will still be believable and accurate.

The lethal dose of ASA is not known, but a single dose of 30 grams is almost always lethal. A standard adult aspirin contains 5 grains or 325 mgs. A grain is about 65 mgs, and 1 gram contains 1,000 mgs. This means that taking 90 aspirin tabs at one time would do almost anyone in. Obviously a much smaller dose would cause the toxic side effects you describe. As few as 6 or 8 tablets at one time could do it, and as many as 20 would cause problems in almost anyone. Taken over several days, as you propose, the levels in the blood would gradually rise as your character took more and more each day, and the toxic effects may not appear for several days.

I would suggest that he take 12 to 20 or so a day (which is not unusual, since people think that aspirin is safe because it's sold over the counter) for the 4 or 5 days you need, and his symptoms would begin on the second or third day and progress from there. If he took 3 or 4 every 6 hours, that would fit the bill. Once he stopped the meds his symptoms would resolve over a day or two, depending upon how severe they were to begin with. To be safe, have him off duty for two days, and then his symptoms should be reduced enough that he could get back to work.

Another point is that at that time many medications were purchased in bulk by the pharmacist and then packaged for the customer. Many pharmacies sold ASA as powders that they folded into pharmacist folds (small paper wrappers). The instructions were usually to take one package every so many hours with water. Or to dissolve it in water and drink it. The important point is that the dose varied widely, depending upon the skill and the weighing equipment of the particular pharmacist. Your detective could take three or four doses five or six times a day.

What Toxic Gas Could Be Used to Kill a Roomful of People?

Q: In the final confrontation scene in my story, forty patients recovering after brain injury and with varying degrees of deficits are trapped in a large dining room with sealed windows and doors. The bad guys are three nurses who see no problem in destroying these patients, who are a costly burden on the medical system. They plan to gas everyone in the room, so I'm looking for a gas that rapidly replaces oxygen and kills quickly. I thought of nitrous dioxide, hydrogen cyanide, and chlorine. Would these work? Any other ideas for my bad guys?

Pauline Alidred

Orange, Massachusetts

A: They must work for an HMO. Cost containment knows no bounds.

Gases can kill by several basic mechanisms. They may be true poisons in that they alter the victim's biochemistry and cause severe illness and death. Cyanide, VX, and sarin are such gases. Some gases are corrosive and damage the lungs, causing them to leak fluid that fills the lungs and prevents breathing. This is called "chemical pulmonary edema," and in this situation the victim basically drowns in these fluids. Chlorine and mustard gas kill in this fashion. Other gases replace oxygen (O_2) in the air, thus lowering the amount of O_2 entering the lungs, and ultimately the bloodstream. This results in a rapid drop of the O_2 level in the blood, and the victim dies of asphyxia. Carbon monoxide (CO) kills this way. Still other gases produce some effect on the victim's physiology that can be lethal. Nitrous oxide (NO_2) causes a rapid drop in the victim's blood pressure, leading to shock and death.

For your scenario I would use NO_2 or CO. Nitrous oxide is "laughing gas," and is used in dental anesthesia. Several of these tanks could be stolen or purchased from a supply house, and the gas could be pumped into the room. Depending upon the size of the room, it could require a few or many tanks. The victims would begin to laugh and get giddy, then become confused and disoriented, collapse, fall into comas, slip into shock, and die. This would take only a very few minutes if the room were small and poorly ventilated (better if it is completely enclosed with no outside air getting in), and if the amount of gas were large. Carbon monoxide is odorless and colorless, comes in tanks, and could also be pumped into the room. The victims would become sleepy, maybe develop slight headaches, become confused and disoriented, fall asleep, slip into comas, and die. This could take anywhere from fifteen minutes to an hour or so, again depending upon the same factors outlined above.

There are many others, but these are available, odorless (so the victims wouldn't know what was happening until it was too late), and would fit your scenario.

When Was Mad Hatter's Disease First Described?

Q: What year did it become common knowledge that mercury was responsible for mad hatter's syndrome, and in what form could a common person obtain mercury or mercury salts during Victorian England? I want the victim to appear to go insane over a period of time before dying.

Tamyra Novinger

A: Hat makers in the nineteenth century began to develop neurological and psychiatric disorders, manifested by weakness, tremors, and personality changes. It was due to the water-soluble mercury nitrate they used to soften and shape animal furs such as beaver pelts. This process was called "felting." Mercury from the felting solution was absorbed through the skin, and the vapors it gave off were inhaled, leading to mercury poisoning.

The first reported recognition of this connection was a study reported by Dr. J. A. Freeman of New Jersey in 1860. Other studies followed over the next sixty years, but it was not until 1941 that mercury was banned in the hat-making industry.

Mercury is also known as quicksilver and was used for many years in the manufacture of mirrors and thermometers. Daniel Fahrenheit (1686–1736) invented the mercury thermometer in 1714, and though the public sale of them has been banned in many areas, they still exist today. In the Victorian period your villain could easily remove some quicksilver from a thermometer and use it for his nefarious deeds. A little added to the victim's food day after day would do it.

Would an Old Bottle of Chloroform Still Be Potent Enough to Render a Person Unconscious?

Q: Was chloroform readily available to physicians in the 1920s? Would a closed bottle of chloroform from that time period still be potent if found today? And would that old plot device of soaking a cloth with chloroform and putting it over someone's face cause them to pass out in a few seconds?

>Hallie Ephron
>
>Coauthor of the Dr. Peter Zak mysteries by G. H. Ephron
>
>www.hallieephron.com

A: Justis von Liebig and French chemist Eugene Souberian discovered chloroform (trichloromethane or methyl trichloride) in 1831. It was first used for anesthesia in Edinburgh, Scotland, by obstetrician James Young Simpson in 1847, and rapidly became a popular surgical anesthetic throughout Europe.

Ether was more common in the United States, owing to its first use as a surgical anesthetic by Dr. Crawford Long in 1842. Chloroform did not receive widespread use in the United States until the beginning of the twentieth century. So yes, it was commonly available in the 1920s.

Chloroform is a volatile liquid, which means it changes rapidly to a gas at room temperature and floats away, like the gasoline you smell at a gas pump. If the bottle in question were very tightly closed it is possible the chloroform could survive for many decades. Or not. But it's at least possible that an old bottle could still be potent.

Yes, soaking a rag works. It may actually take a minute or so, and not seconds, but it works. In fact, that is exactly how it was given through much of its history as a surgical anesthetic.

What Happens to a Person Who Attempts Suicide by Drinking a Chlorine Bleach Product?

Q: One of my characters drinks a hefty amount of chlorine bleach in a suicide attempt. What might happen to her? What pain will she experience? Will she vomit? How much time does she have? If someone got her to the hospital in time, what long-term effects might it have on her?

A: Most chlorine bleaches contain sodium hypochlorite, which is a chemical irritant. That means that it is not truly a poison in the sense that arsenic is, but rather that it irritates or burns any and all tissues it contacts. It will burn and redden the skin and eyes. If swallowed, the same thing happens to the mouth, esophagus (swallowing tube), and stomach.

With ingestion she would sense a burning pain in her mouth, throat, and chest, would become nauseated, and would likely vomit. If the bleach was concentrated enough and/or if the contact with the esophagus and stomach was long enough, bleeding could occur. It would be unlikely that she would die, however, since vomiting would occur fairly quickly in most cases.

She could choke and aspirate the bleach into her lungs. Aspiration is simply the inhaling of any substance into the lungs. This could occur while drinking the liquid or during vomiting. If chlorine bleach enters the lungs it can cause severe damage and could lead to pulmonary edema (lungs filled with water). This occurs because the bleach burns the lung tissues, which causes them to leak fluid into the alveoli (air sacs) of the lungs. She would become very short of breath, with severe coughing, and could develop respiratory failure and die.

In the ER they would give her fluids and, if she aspirated, steroids (such as intravenous Decadron) to lessen the damage to the lungs. She would receive oxygen to help her breathe and antibiotics to hopefully prevent a secondary infection of the damaged lungs. If she developed pulmonary edema and respiratory failure she might require a ventilator for a while. She could recover with no long-term effects or could be left with residual lung and stomach problems.

Can Injecting Drain Cleaner into My Victim Cause Death?

Q: For my story I have an odd question about a very deranged killer. Would injecting 10cc of drain cleaner into a person kill them? What would happen to them?

Edward R. Johnstun

Blanding, Utah

A: Drano and other drain-cleaning products are highly corrosive. Check out the warning label on any of these products. Scary stuff. If swallowed they will severely damage the mouth, esophagus, and stomach, and if aspirated, the lungs. The latter injury is why inducing vomiting in those who ingest these liquids is not a bright idea. If they aspirated any of the vomited material, the lungs could be severely damaged.

If injected intramuscularly (IM, or into the muscles), it would cause a great deal of pain and local damage, but might not kill the victim. At least not quickly. But if it were injected intravenously (IV), it would have the same corrosive effects on the blood vessels, and probably on the heart.

Ten ccs should do your character in. Painfully, but quickly. Let's say your villain injected the cleaner into one of the victim's arm veins. A fiery pain would travel up the arm, and if the cleaner reached the heart in sufficient concentration it would irritate it, which could lead to deadly arrhythmias (changes in heart rhythm). The victim would react violently to the pain, but when the heart rhythm changed to something deadly, he would collapse and die. This could take seconds or minutes.

What Was the Treatment for a Heroin Overdose in the 1980s?

Q: How is heroin overdose treated in the ER? What drugs or interventional procedures would be implemented? Could the treatment actually begin in the field or ambulance? Would these interventions be available in the mid 1980s and early 1990s?

Jannice Genaux
Waco, Texas

A: The treatment for a heroin overdose is the same now as it was in the 1980s.

Heroin is an opiate, which means it is derived from the opium poppy. It is a powerful depressant, which causes sleepiness, lethargy, and coma. If too much is taken, heroin depresses the respiratory centers of the brain and the user can stop breathing and die of asphyxia.

The first step in treatment is to reestablish breathing. A face mask or an endotracheal (ET) tube (plastic tube placed into the trachea, or windpipe) with an attached Ambu bag (an air-filled bladder that pumps air into the mask as it is squeezed rhythmically), is used to pump oxygen into the victim's lungs (respiration). This would be started in the field by the paramedics, and continued during transport in the ambulance.

In the emergency room the victim would be placed on a ventilator, an intravenous (IV) line would be started, and Narcan would be given IV. Narcan is a drug that blocks the depressing effects of the heroin and other opiates almost instantly. The victim would likely begin breathing and wake up, and might even become combative and hard to control. The ET tube could then be removed. However, the ordeal is not over. The victim must be monitored very closely for recurring sleepiness, coma, and respiratory depression, and the Narcan may have to be given several times over the first hour or so until the heroin is metabolized (broken down by body enzymes). Large amounts of IV fluids would be given to "flush" the kidneys.

If the victim were treated quickly and effectively, he would do well. If any delay occurred, and the victim was without respirations for several minutes, he could be left with permanent brain damage.

How Long Can a Balloon Filled with Heroin Remain Intact Within a "Mule's" Stomach?

Q: How long might one of those plastic bags full of heroin or cocaine survive intact in a drug mule's stomach before they have to worry about the bag bursting or leaking?

Brian Thornton
Seattle, Washington
Author of *101 Things You Didn't Know About Lincoln*

A: "Drug mules" are people who swallow packets of drugs in order to sneak them through Customs. Most use either balloons or condoms. The transit time of the GI tract is about twenty-four hours. That is, from intake to excretion is about a day. So the mule has about twenty-four hours to complete his journey. After that the balloons are passed and collected. I don't know who gets that job in the illegal drug industry hierarchy.

Stomach acids, digestive enzymes, and the peristaltic motion of the bowels work to break down any food that enter the GI tract. Drug-filled balloons get the same treatment. Will the condom/balloon survive the journey? Either it will or it won't. There is no way to predict it. Fortunately, most do come through intact. If not, the mule is a goner. A condom full of heroin or cocaine will kill very quickly if it breaks or leaks any significant amount.

The condoms/balloons are visible on X-rays and fluoroscopy, so if a mule is suspected, the Drug Enforcement Administration (DEA) guys will simply run them under a fluoroscope, and bingo! They will then give the mule a laxative—usually something like magnesium citrate—and collect the evidence. I imagine rookies get this job.

So the drugs would be in the mule for only about twenty-four hours, thirty-six to forty-eight at the outside, and they could rupture or leak at any time. I guess you would call this Colombian roulette.

Can a Death-Row Inmate Be Saved After Receiving a Lethal Injection?

Q: When a prisoner is given a lethal injection, is it possible to save them if another drug is given in time?

Lee Goldberg

Los Angeles, California

Author of the Diagnosis Murder and Monk series

www.leegoldberg.com

A: Yes.

Lethal injection consists of three drugs, not one: a sedative such as sodium pentothal, a muscle paralytic such as succinylcholine (Anectine) or vecuronium bromide (Norcuron), and potassium chloride (KCl). They are given intravenously (IV) in succession. The sedative and paralytic drugs vary, but potassium chloride is essentially universal. The sedative puts the victim to sleep, so the process is painless. The paralytic drug paralyzes all the muscles of the body, including those used for breathing, and potassium chloride stops the heart.

Simply breathing for the victim will prevent death from the first two drugs. An Ambu bag (a football-shaped device that will deliver a breath of air every time it is squeezed) attached to a face mask or an endotracheal (ET) tube (passed through the nose or mouth and into the windpipe) will suffice, and is easily used. Or a ventilator can be attached to the ET tube. Respiration is supported until the drugs are metabolized (broken down) by the body. This may take an hour or more, but if done properly the victim would survive without problem.

The KCl is more problematic. Since the heart will stop immediately upon injection, CPR must be instituted quickly. CPR consists of the above breathing measures plus external cardiac massage (pushing on the chest to compress the heart in a rhythmic fashion, which simulates the pumping of the heart and circulates the blood through the body). While this is underway an IV injection of a mixture of glucose and insulin and/or calcium chloride may reverse the effect of the potassium. It's complex biochemistry, but the net effect is that the heart should begin to beat once again. These drugs may have to be repeated over the next hour as needed, but eventually the body excretes the excess potassium, and all is once again okay.

So, to save someone who has received a triple-drug lethal injection, you must support respiration, begin CPR, and give a mixture of glucose and insulin and/or calcium chloride IV.

What Drug or Drugs Might Be Given to Someone to Cause Depression and Suicide?

Q: I need to know what common and available drug or combination of drugs could be secretly given to one of my characters and cause severe depression and provoke him to commit suicide. The drug can be given over a few days or weeks if necessary. In my story the victim is already on one drug, but it's the surreptitious giving of a second drug that causes the problems. Any suggestions?

A: Drugs that have psychiatric effects are given the general term of psychotropic drugs. These come in many flavors and are used to elevate moods; to ease depression; to calm the overly active; to treat delusions, hallucinations, and other manifestations of schizophrenia and other serious psychiatric disorders; and for many other psychiatric ills.

All of these medications have a laundry list of side effects and unexpected reactions that are often unpredictable in any given individual. One person may become depressed, even suicidal, another may become hyperactive, another may develop paranoid delusions, and yet another may become aggressive and dangerous to themselves and others. One truth about all psychoactive drugs is that they can sometimes cause what they are intended to cure. That is, a drug that is supposed to help depression might make it worse. A classic example is Ritalin. In a normal person it will tend to act like speed or an upper. Yet in children with one of the hyperactive disorders it usually calms them. The bottom line is that each of us has different brain chemistry, so chemicals added to the mix will behave differently in each of us.

For the scenario you describe, any combination of antidepressants or medications with depressive side effects could lead to further depression and suicide in your intended victim. The problem is that your killer can't predict that, so it will be a matter of "luck" as to whether the combination will work, and if so over what time frame. Too many variables for your story, I suspect.

But you might consider a different, nonsuicidal type of death. If the victim was already depressed and was taking a class of antidepressants known as monoamine oxidase inhibitors, or MAOIs for short, he would be vulnerable to the action of some other drugs and foods.

MAOIs alter the chemistry of the brain by blocking the enzyme monoamine oxidase, which normally breaks down norepinephrine and other neurotransmitters in the brain. It's complex biochemistry, and it's not necessary to explain, except that a person on an MAOI must not take some other meds and must avoid certain foods. If not, a hypertensive crisis could ensue. In this situation the blood pressure (BP) abruptly shoots up, and the person can suffer a stroke, heart attack, and death.

Common MAOIs are: Nardil (phenelzine), Parnate (tranylcypromine), and Marplan (isocarboxazid).

Drugs that can cause a hypertensive reaction when taken in conjunction with one of these MAOIs are: amphetamines and all types of "diet pills," Flexeril (cyclobenzaprine), Prozac (fluoxetine), Paxil (paroxetine), Zoloft (sertraline), Demerol (meperidine), and any of the tricyclate antidepressants such as Elavil (amitriptyline), Sinequan (doxepin), and Tofranil (imipramine). There are many others, but these are common medications.

Foods to avoid are those that are high in the amino acid tyramine, such as certain cheeses, fava beans, smoked or pickled meats, fermented sausages (bologna, pepperoni, salami, and summer sausage), alcohol, caffeinated drinks such as coffee, tea, and colas, and chocolate. The list is much longer, but this gives you the idea and some choices.

If your character was secretly given or was taking one of the MAOIs for some mild depression, your villain could then slip him an amphetamine or a diet pill or a couple of Paxils and wait. In a few minutes to an hour or so his BP would shoot up, he would develop a severe headache, blurred vision, and shortness of breath, and then he'd collapse. He could or could not have a seizure with this. The elevated BP damages the brain, and may even cause bleeding into the brain. This would be called a hypertensive hemorrhagic stroke. That means that the stroke resulted from bleeding (hemorrhagic) into the brain due to an elevated BP (hypertensive).

What Drug Would Render an Inmate Work-Crew Guard Unconscious?

Q: I'm working on a scene where three inmates at the county jail are on roadside cleanup duty, followed by a county vehicle. The guard/driver is drinking coffee and eating brownies baked by the jailed chef, while he supposedly keeps an eye on his charges. I'd like the driver to doze off, allowing the three to get away. Would marijuana baked into the brownies work? If not, what would?

Cynthia Riggs
Martha's Vineyard, Massachusetts
www.cynthiariggs.com

A: Marijuana could work, but it might also make him run to the 7-Eleven for a Snickers. It does have sedative effects but probably not powerful enough for your needs. And the coffee wouldn't help your guys get away either. I'd suggest any of the common sedatives such as Valium, Ativan, or Xanax. These are all tranquilizers and come in pill form. Three or four tablets of any of these dissolved in a drink or crushed and added to food such as brownies would work. Each of these would take about thirty minutes or so to work, and the victim would be out for from two to six hours, depending upon the amount given and many other factors.

Another good choice would be chloral hydrate. When mixed with any alcohol it is a very powerful sedative, and the combination of these two was the original Mickey Finn, or Mickey. It works very well alone, too. It comes as a child's sedative by the trade name Noctec. It is a liquid, and a couple of tablespoons added to a drink would do the trick.

There are, of course, many others, but these are easily available since they reside in many people's medicine cabinets. And prisoners are usually very clever and can get all kinds of things into the jail, including prescription medications.

Any of these would be a more reliable and predictable sedative than marijuana and would be better for your needs.

How Does "Truth Serum" Work?

Q: One of my characters, a twenty-one-year-old woman, is subjected to an interrogation with a "truth serum" such as sodium pentothal. My research says that the subject would have a reaction somewhat similar to being drunk. True? And if she were overdosed with the drug what would happen, and how could my hero save her from death?

> James Lee (writing as Destron)
> Philippines
> www.fictionpress.com/~destron

A: Truth serums are simply sedatives, and it is this sedative effect that makes them useful in interrogations. One interrogative technique that works is sleep deprivation, since this breaks down the person's defenses, slows their mental functions, and causes them to say things they otherwise wouldn't. But this takes time. Two or three days, perhaps more. Sedatives, such as sodium pentothal, bring about the same mental effects in a matter of minutes. The victim is sleepy and confused, her judgment is impaired, her defenses are weakened, her mental processes are slowed, and she says things that she shouldn't.

As with any sedative, too much will lead to loss of consciousness, coma, a cessation of breathing, and death. To save her your hero would need to call for medical help and attempt to arouse her. If she stopped breathing before help arrived, he would have to use mouth-to-mouth respiration to breathe for her until the cavalry came. Or until the drug's effects wore off, which could be several hours.

Can Tampering with an Elderly Woman's Medications Cause Her Death?

Q: I have an elderly character whose brother is trying to kill her. She takes multiple pills every day, one of which is for her high blood pressure and another for her heart. If either of these pills was replaced by a placebo (and she didn't notice), would that eventually kill her?

Karen Elliott (writing as K. Grant Elliott)
Albuquerque, New Mexico

A: This is one of the easiest murders to disguise. Why? Because improperly taken medications kill people more frequently than most people realize. And older people screw up their meds—take too much or not enough—all the time. It can go either way. Either withholding needed meds or giving too much can cause death. Withholding is usually less predictable than overdosing, but it will work.

Let's say your victim has high blood pressure (HBP) and is taking HBP meds such as a calcium channel blocker (common ones would be Norvasc or Procardia) or an ACE inhibitor (common ones are Vasotec, Zestril, and Prinivil). Withholding them for a day or two could lead to a rapid rise in her blood pressure (BP) and cause a stroke or heart attack. Maybe. It's not predictable, so your killer couldn't be sure that this would work. On the other hand, giving a large dose at once could cause the BP to drop rapidly and lead to a heart attack or cardiac arrest. If the killer crumbled several pills in the victim's food or drink, and she took this along with her usual dose, she could die anywhere from thirty minutes to two hours or so after taking the extra, hidden dose.

And if the ME were to test the levels of the drugs in the body (he probably wouldn't unless he had a high level of suspicion that something was amiss), he would find either a high or a low level and assume the victim was taking her medications incorrectly. He might simply write off the death as an accidental overdose of prescription drugs. As I said, this happens not infrequently.

The one way the ME might determine that something was wrong would be if you use the overdose scenario. Most accidental overdoses by elderly people come about because they begin taking a once-a-day medication twice or three times a day. If so the levels of the drug in the body can rise over several days to deadly levels. With toxicological testing these very high levels in the blood could be found easily. High blood levels would be found whether the victim took the overdose over several days or took a handful of pills all at once, so this wouldn't help the ME distinguish a slow overdose from a fast one.

But if the ME also tested the victim's stomach contents and found very high levels of unabsorbed drug in the victim's stomach, he could conclude that the victim had not been taking too many pills accidentally over several days, but rather that she had taken several pills at once. Though still possible, this would less likely be an accident. Could be, or could be a suicide, but he would at least have to consider homicide. You might be able to use this if you ultimately want this event to lead to the killer's capture.

What Drug Available in the 1960s Would Cause Severe Intoxication in My Character?

Q: I have a character who needs to intoxicate a man so she can sleep with him, or at least fool him into believing she did. He's not one to tip the bottle. The story is set in the Deep South in the late 1960s, and my character is uneducated, poor, not very sophisticated, and pretty dense. Does the aspirin in the Coke thing work, or was that an old wives' tale? What else might she use?

Kathleen Antrim
Author of *Capital Offense*
www.kathleenantrim.com

A: No, aspirin and Coke won't work. That's an old legend. Her best bet is a sedative with or without alcohol. She could put the sedative in a cola or fruit drink, or in some spicy food to hide its slight bitterness. Common ones available in the 1960s would be a barbiturate (Seconal, Tuinal, phenobarbital), chloral hydrate, and paregoric, which is tincture of opium. The barbiturates are capsules, which can be opened and the powder dissolved into food or drink, and the other two are liquids. Two or three capsules or a couple of teaspoons of the liquids should do the trick.

He would get "drunk," silly, stupid, sleepy, and compliant, and finally would fall asleep. He may not remember much, which is what you want.

What Drugs Were Available During the Medieval Period That Could Render a Character Unconscious?

Q: My story is set during the medieval period. My main character needs to render another character unconscious for several hours. I thought of asphyxiation, but the victim recovers in too short a time. The only other thing I can think of is the classic "hitting someone over the head," though I think that only works in movies.

A: You're right. The knockout blow that leaves the character unconscious for the rest of the movie is a Hollywood deal, and has little basis in real life. Think of all the boxers you've seen knocked out on TV. They're up and complaining about a lucky punch in about half a minute. And this is after a blow from someone trained to knock people out.

This means that neither strangulation nor a knockout blow will work for your scenario. With asphyxiation, unless there is permanent brain damage, the person would wake up very quickly after the constricting device (hands or ligature) was removed. The same is true for a blow to the head. Again, unless permanent brain damage occurred, the person may be out for several seconds or minutes, even up to twenty or thirty minutes, but not for hours.

What you will need is a sedative of some type. During the medieval period both alcohol and opium were available. A mixture would be particularly powerful. Opium came as a white powder or mixed with water to make a liquid. It is very bitter but could be masked by spicy food. If your victim were given several drinks and a little opium he could be out for an hour or up to eight or ten hours, depending upon the dose.

How Quickly Could a Combination of Xanax and Alcohol Kill My Character?

Q: I have a short story in progress, and I need some help with my chosen poison. How long would it take for fifteen Xanax tablets (crushed and added to a rum and Diet Coke) to kill a woman who weighed 110 pounds? I'm hoping it would be quick, maybe five minutes or so. Am I dreaming?

Jerrilyn Farmer
Los Angeles, California
Author of *Desperately Seeking Sushi* and many other
Madeline Bean mysteries

A: Xanax (alprazolam) alone won't do it. Rum makes it work. Xanax is actually a fairly safe drug, with a wide safety margin. She would have to be given fifty or hundred tablets to do her in. But, if mixed with alcohol, ten or so might do it. It would be best if she were already intoxicated before the Xanax was given. And after several drinks she might not notice the medicinal taste of the Xanax in the doctored drink.

She would become giddy, intoxicated, and then lethargic and off balance. Her speech would slur, she would stagger, and would finally slip into a coma, stop breathing, and die from asphyxiation. If she had already had a few drinks, this entire process could happen over fifteen minutes or so if the Xanax-laced drink was taken on an empty stomach. Or an hour or more if she had eaten recently, since this would slow down the absorption of both the Xanax and the alcohol into the bloodstream. She could then stop breathing and die over the next ten to twenty minutes. This is extremely variable. So overall your scenario will work. I would suggest lengthening the time from five minutes to fifteen or more, if you can.

When Do the Initial Symptoms of a Rattlesnake Bite Appear, and What Are the Long-Term Problems Associated with a Bite?

Q: How long after receiving a bite from a medium–size Western Diamondback rattler will symptoms appear? In particular, how long might it take for a nonfatal bite to cause a victim to lose consciousness?

Assuming it is a matter of a few hours before any treatment, and that antitoxins are not available, what's a reasonable time for a full recovery? What kind of permanent but invisible damage might result?

A: There are approximately 120 species of snakes in the United States, but only about twenty are poisonous. Every state has at least one venomous snake except Maine, Alaska, and Hawaii. All of the bad guys are pit vipers, except for the coral snake, which ranges throughout the southeastern United States. Pit vipers derive their name from the small heat-sensing "pit" near the eyes, which helps them locate prey. The deadliest of the pit vipers are the Diamondback rattlers, both Eastern and Western. So your character's run-in will be with a bad one.

With modern treatments (such as antivenin), and with more rapid transport of victims to the hospital, only five or six deaths occur out of the seven thousand to eight thousand snakebites per year. In your scenario none of these modern benefits are available, so your character will need luck and at least some treatment. Did I mention luck?

Ninety-eight percent of bites are to the extremities—legs, arms, and hands. The most common symptoms are pain, swelling, and bruising in the area of the bite, nausea, vomiting, and collapse, with loss of consciousness. The victim would appear pale, cold, and clammy. These symptoms may have nothing to do with the toxin, but rather result from the absolute terror that a snakebite generates in the victim. Of course, these may also result from the venom.

The severity of the injury, the rapidity of symptom onset, and the ultimate outcome depend upon the type and age of the snake (often the young ones possess a more concentrated venom); the location, depth, and amount of venom injected (the big ones have longer fangs); and the size, weight, and general health of the victim.

The signs and symptoms of snakebite are divided into local and systemic (total body) reactions. Snake venom is a complex fluid. It typically has several proteases (enzymes that break down proteins—basically, digest them), which can lead to severe damage to the tissues near the bite. These can be so severe that surgical debridement (removal of dead tissue) and even amputation may be necessary. Also, infection can occur in the injured tissues, which can in and of itself be serious and deadly. This was particularly true in the preantibiotic era of the nineteenth and early twentieth centuries.

Local effects may be fang marks, pain, swelling, redness, the appearance of bullae (blisters), lymphangitis (red streaks up the extremity), and painful knots in the axilla (armpit) or groin. The knots are swollen lymph nodes. These symptoms and signs begin immediately and progress if not treated.

Systemic problems result from other components of the venom. These tend to appear shortly after envenomation and progress over several hours. The systemic symptoms and signs include nausea; vomiting; numbness and tingling of the hands, face, and feet; weakness; a metallic taste in the mouth; shortness of breath; confusion; coma; and shock. Confusion and loss of consciousness may occur within minutes or several hours, depending upon the degree of envenomation. The blood may clot or hemolyze (break down), and can lead to kidney damage or death, or at least to significant anemia. The blood pressure will be very low, and the pulse very weak. Death can follow. Or, as in your scenario, the victim could survive.

Rural treatment would be cutting open the wound; letting it bleed freely for several minutes; wrapping and elevating the extremity; comfort measures; and prayer. The old treatment of sucking out the venom is often done but is not recommended, since the person performing this procedure may actually poison himself.

With a significant envenomation it may take several days for him to be up and around, and a week or so before he regains all his strength. He may be completely normal, or he could have a nasty scar around the site of the bite, a residual from the damage done by the proteases. He could also have long-term neurological defects such as weakness and/or numbness of the extremity bitten.

Would a Rattlesnake Bite to the Carotid Artery Kill Quickly?

Q: In my story a Pacific rattlesnake (*Crotalus viridis oreganos*) strikes a twenty-year-old woman who weighs about 110 pounds. She is crawling under a building and is struck in the carotid artery. How long would it take for her to die?

Norm Benson
Lower Lake, California

A: When a snake bites it injects venom into the penetrated tissues, usually a foot, leg, arm, or hand. Rattlesnake venom contains several toxic substances, some of which cause local injury and others that cause systemic (throughout the body) injuries.

Local injuries include bruising, swelling, and with some venoms a "digestion" of the surrounding tissues. Components of the venom act as enzymes and break down the proteins in human tissues. This is similar to the digestive enzymes that work within our own GI tract.

Systemic injuries include a drop in blood pressure (BP) with shock, damage to blood cells, and damage to the clotting proteins in the blood (these are the proteins that make blood clot), which leads to severe bleeding. Some snake toxins also damage the brain and the nerves, which causes confusion, disorientation, weakness, numbness and tingling of the extremities, coma, depression of the respiratory center, cessation of breathing, and death.

With limb envenomation (toxin injection) the local symptoms begin in ten to thirty minutes and the systemic ones in one to twelve hours. This varies a great deal depending upon the size, age, and health of the victim and the degree of envenomation from the bite. This in turn depends upon the species, size, and venom concentration of the snake involved.

But if the venom were injected into the carotid artery, all these symptoms would come on within minutes, and death could take as little as three or four minutes. Could be longer, could be less. This means that you have a broad range of times for your story. I'd make death occur somewhere between two and twenty minutes after the bite, and you'll be okay.

Does Aconite (Monkshood) Make an Effective Poison, and Can It Be Found by the ME at Autopsy?

Q: A seventy-year-old man dies from ingesting aconite (monkshood) poison that was baked into some food, and an autopsy is performed because no one was present when he died. Will the ME find this poison in the general autopsy or just assume he died of heart problems or some other old-age problem? In addition, is it possible the lab could detect the poison in some of the uneaten food? I want readers to know this was an intentional poisoning from the start and not something he could have accidentally come into contact with.

Tammy Coulter

Madison, Alabama

A: Aconite (monkshood, wolfsbane, friar's cap, blue rocket) is a plant about three feet tall with dark green leaves and dark blue flowers. It contains several dangerous alkaloids, including aconitine, aconine, sparteine, and ephedrine. The name wolfsbane dates to medieval times, when arrows were dipped into the plant's juice prior to wolf hunting. The same technique was used during warfare.

It was used for a wide variety of medical problems, and indeed is still sold today as a homeopathic remedy, as a diuretic, and as a diaphoretic (to cause sweating). The symptoms of an overdose include weakness; cold and clammy skin; shortness of breath; nausea; vomiting; numbness and tingling of the tongue, mouth, and skin; giddiness; a staggering gait; and, if enough is given, coma and death.

In the scenario you outline it is likely that the ME would assign the death to a natural occurrence such as a heart attack or a cardiac arrhythmia, since these are common causes of death in elderly men. Why would he even consider poisoning? Unless the situation or a witness suggested that poisoning was involved, he wouldn't likely do expensive and time-consuming toxicological testing. He has a budget, and contrary to *CSI*, it is not unlimited. He must justify expenses, and thus would not perform expensive testing without good cause. But if he did, he could find the toxins in the victim's blood and stomach contents, and also in any food that contained the toxin.

This means you can have it either way. The ME signs the death off as a natural event, and the killer gets away with it, or he becomes suspicious and does the testing and finds the true cause of death. Either will work.

Can Antifreeze Ingestion Kill an Alcoholic?

Q: My story involves the murder of an alcoholic woman. Could an alcoholic drink a beverage laced with antifreeze without realizing it? Would she taste the antifreeze? How would the antifreeze kill the alcoholic?

Joanna Paxinou
Marina, California

A: The major toxic ingredient in most antifreeze solutions is ethylene glycol. For some reason antifreeze (along with turpentine and paint thinners) is a favorite beverage of alcoholics when they can't get ethanol. Since antifreeze causes intoxication it is seen as a substitute for ethanol. This means that your character would probably drink it, and may do so even if she knew what it was. Unfortunately it is also deadly.

The symptoms of ethylene glycol intake include nausea, vomiting, confusion, disorientation, slurred speech, a staggering gait, and, if enough is consumed, seizures, coma, and death. These same symptoms are seen with alcohol intoxication. But the real problems with ethylene glycol come from the chemical reactions it undergoes in the body, where it is broken down into several compounds, the most important being oxalic acid. This acid causes the deposition of oxalate crystals in the brain and kidneys, which results in irreparable damage and death. At autopsy the ME will find the oxalate crystals in the tubules of the kidney.

What Drug Could My Character Use to Make Someone Violently Ill but Not Kill Them?

Q: Is there an herbal emetic or some other tasteless or almost tasteless substance that would make someone vomit violently but not kill them. I prefer something "herby," since my character will sprinkle it in an electric teapot and let the tea maker do the rest. The tea drinker, my protagonist, drinks herbal tea, so a few leafy flakes or dust in a cup of tea would not be noticed.

A: There are many herbs that can cause nausea and vomiting and, if enough is taken, can be fatal. A smaller dose will make your protagonist sick, and a larger one could kill her. Any of these could work for your scenario:

> **Ipecac:** This is actually used in hospitals and ERs in a liquid form to induce vomiting in drug overdoses. It has a distinct medicinal taste, which could be masked with flavorful or spicy food. A teaspoon or two could be added to a strong tea, and perhaps could pass unnoticed. Also, since ipecac is derived from the berries and plant juices of the *Cephaelis ipecacuanha* plant, you could dry and crumble some of the plant material or seeds, or could make a tea by steeping the plant or berries for several minutes. This tea could be added to the victim's herbal tea. It causes nausea and vomiting in about ten minutes, and also causes the victim to experience shortness of breath, dizziness, and a rapid heartbeat. In higher doses it can lead to loss of consciousness, coma, and death.

> **Castor bean:** The toxin here is ricin, which has been in the news a lot lately as a possible bioterror weapon. Castor beans are very toxic, so a single bean is enough to make someone very ill, and two or three would kill most people. Intact beans are not harmful, since the outer shell is tough and resists digestion. However, if the beans are cut or crushed the toxin is readily accessible. As with ipecac your character could crush one of the beans and add it to the victim's dried tea, or could steep a bean or two and add the resulting liquid to the victim's tea. The victim would quickly develop nausea, vomiting, diarrhea, shortness of breath, and weakness.

> **Oleander:** This plant is very common and easily obtained. All parts of the plant are toxic, so steeping some leaves, stems,

and/or roots would produce a toxic tea. The victim would suffer nausea, vomiting, diarrhea, sweating, and shortness of breath, and if enough were given, coma and death.

Foxglove: This is the plant from which digitalis, an important cardiac medication, is derived. It's also a deadly toxin. The toxins in foxglove are predominantly the glycosides digitoxin and digitonin. These cause nausea, vomiting, shortness of breath, blurred vision, alteration of color vision so that the world takes on a yellowish hue, and cardiac arrhythmias (changes in the normal rhythm of the heart), which can be deadly.

There are many other candidates, but any of these would work.

If a Severely Allergic Person Used Outdated or Altered Medication, Would They Die from an Inadequately Treated Allergic Reaction?

Q: My desperate villain wants to substitute an outdated EpiPen for the newer one the victim carries. He plans to pull the hero act, give her the injection himself, and leave the empty injector with the victim so that it will look as if she forgot to replace it and the outdated medication did not work. I've heard that two years is about the life expectancy of the EpiPen, so if it is older than that does it lose its effects? She is severely allergic to peanuts, and he plans to give her a snack that contains hidden peanuts. He will also feed her a couple of glasses of wine, so that she doesn't sense the allergic reaction too quickly. After the injection he plans to slip away and rejoin friends, so he'll have an alibi by the time the body is found a few minutes later. Would a two-year-old pen still save her life or would my villain's plan work?

Nancy J. Sheedy
Frederick, Maryland

A: EpiPen is a prepackaged automatic injector that delivers a dose of epinephrine, which is often life saving when an acute allergic reaction takes place. We call these severe and deadly allergic reactions "anaphylaxis." Individuals who are severely allergic to things such as peanuts and other foods, bees, and almost anything else often carry an EpiPen.

If properly stored in a refrigerated place, EpiPens can last for many years, and if not, less. There is no exact date at which it will quit working. At best its effects would be weakened and unpredictable after the expiration date. But it could still work. A wise criminal would not depend upon this unknown. It would be better for him to tamper with the injector's contents by diluting it with water, and thus making it less potent. Of course, the spent injector could be tested, and this dilution could be discovered, but this would not likely occur. Why? Because people with allergies occasionally die in spite of proper treatment. EpiPen is not a cure-all, and sometimes it isn't enough even if the dose is proper.

The general rule is that the more severe the allergic reaction the more rapidly it appears. Ingested allergens take longer to react than do injected ones such as bee stings, where the reaction can be almost immediate. In your victim the reaction would likely occur within minutes, but you could allow twenty to thirty minutes at the outside and still be on safe ground.

I would suggest that he simply replace her EpiPen with one that he had tampered with, give her the snack with the "hidden" peanuts (actually a little peanut oil will work), and he can be long gone before she eats the snack. She would then give herself the injection, which would not work, and she would die within a very few minutes. Even if other people were around and the paramedics were called, she could die before they arrived if her allergy was very severe. This would solve your timeline problem, since your villain would set the stage and then disappear. No one would suspect him unless someone besides the victim knew that he had given her the peanut oil–laced snack. With this sequence the wine is not necessary.

Can an Injection of Potassium Kill a Hospitalized Patient Quickly?

Q: This is my story scenario: A 450-pound female patient in otherwise good health is in the preop waiting area of a hospital. She will be given a preop medication through her IV. It will really be KCl, and she dies suddenly. It looks like a heart attack brought on by her excess weight. How much KCl will she have to get to kill her? How long will it take for her to die? Is there any way that the coroner might miss the real cause of death? Would they always do an autopsy in this situation?

Kim Calabrese, RN

Buffalo, New York

A: Potassium chloride (KCl) is the third drug given in lethal-injection executions. It will stop the heart immediately. The dose required depends upon the rate of infusion. When we need to give a patient intravenous (IV) KCl, we avoid giving more than 10 milliequivalents (meqs) per hour. In true emergencies we might give up to 15 meqs per hour, but very rarely any faster than this. If given by rapid IV injection, as little as 10 meqs might do your character in. Thirty or 40 for sure. The victim would suffer a stoppage of the heart in a matter of seconds, and the death would indeed look like a heart attack or a cardiac arrhythmia (a deadly change in the heart's rhythm).

One caveat is that KCl burns like crazy when injected through an IV line. Unless sedated, which might be the situation in the preop area, the victim could cry out. For the few seconds before things faded to black, that is. Another way to avoid the victim reacting would be for her to have a central IV line. This is one that is not in an arm vein, but rather is passed up through an arm vein and into or near the right atrium of the heart. KCl injected through such a line would cause no burning.

In any unexplained hospital death the ME or coroner would be notified. He may or may not get involved in the case. If the treating M.D. says the victim died of a heart attack or cardiac arrhythmia, and is willing to sign the death certificate stating that this is the case, the ME might accept this. This would be the end of it, and your killer would have gotten away with murder.

But if the treating M.D. was unsure of the cause of death, the ME would most likely take the case, and would perform an autopsy. In these types of in-hospital deaths, none of the IV lines or other medical devices are removed after death by the hospital personnel, but rather the victim is shipped to the coroner with everything in place. The reason is that the invasive devices that were used in a particular patient may be part of the cause of death. As in this case.

The ME may or may not find the cause of death, however. Thirty or 40 meqs of KCl would not likely elevate the blood potassium level to a large extent, since this amount of potassium would be quickly diluted throughout the body, and would be taken up by the body's cells rapidly. He could find high KCl levels in the IV tubing, so a strong flush of the line with saline after the KCl is given would be wise. If so, there may be no evidence of the true cause of death, and it may be written off as a routine lethal cardiac arrhythmia.

Could My Character Use Cyanide Added to a Contact Lens Solution to Kill Another Character?

Q: I have a scenario in which my victim dies from poison—either cyanide or strychnine—which has been added to her contact lens saline solution. Which is better, cyanide or strychnine? How soon after inserting the lens into her eye would she die? How much of the poison needs to be added to the solution?

Maggie King
Richmond, Virginia

A: I'd go with cyanide, since it is absorbed through the skin, whereas strychnine is more powerful if swallowed. And it takes only a tiny amount of cyanide to do the trick.

Cyanide is quick, nasty, and effective. It is what we call a "metabolic poison" because it basically shuts down the ability of all the body's cells to use oxygen. The red blood cells (RBCs) cannot carry oxygen to the tissues, and the tissue cells of the body can't use the oxygen anyway. It is as if all the oxygen were removed from the body instantly. This process is immediate and profound and leads to death in one to ten minutes, depending on the dosage.

Symptoms would begin almost immediately in the delivery method you have chosen. The symptoms are rapid breathing, shortness of breath, dizziness, flushing, nausea, vomiting, and loss of consciousness, maybe seizure activity, and then death. So the victim would develop sudden severe shortness of breath, a flushed face, perhaps clutch at her chest, collapse to the floor, and die, with or without having a seizure in the process. Her skin would appear very pink, and if she hit her head or scraped an elbow in her fall and bled, the blood would be a noticeably bright cherry red. This is due to a chemical reaction between the cyanide and the hemoglobin molecules in the RBCs, which produces cyanohemoglobin, a bright red chemical.

Potassium cyanide (KCN) and sodium cyanide (NaCN) are white powders with a faint bitter almond smell, which most people do not notice. In fact, the ability to sense this odor is genetically determined. Some people can, and others can't. Both KCN and NaCN dissolve readily in water and saline, so either could be easily added to your victim's contact solution.

One caveat: Your killer must be careful in handling these chemicals. They are readily absorbed through the skin and could do in your bad guy. Rubber gloves would be wise.

KCN and NaCN are used commercially in metal recovery such as extracting gold or silver from their ores, and in electroplating such metals as gold, silver, copper, and platinum. They could be pilfered from a jewelry or metal-plating company, and are also sold by several chemical supply firms.

In your story the powder could be dissolved in the eye-cleaner fluid, and when the victim squirted it into her eyes or soaked her contacts in it and slipped them into her eyes, she would collapse and die very quickly.

What Chemical Could Make a Cigarette Toxic?

Q: In my political thriller the bad guys try to kill a newspaper reporter who is uncovering their nefarious activities. Since he smokes I plan to have another character approach him in a bar and offer him a cigarette to which some toxin has been added. But what? I want the substance to be potentially deadly, but I want my reporter to become ill yet survive. Any ideas?

Kathleen Antrim
Author of *Capital Offense*
www.kathleenantrim.com

A: Adding a poison to a cigarette that is then inhaled along with the tobacco smoke is a diabolical idea, and is relatively easy to pull off. What smoker wouldn't accept a free smoke? Particularly at today's prices. Several toxins could fit your requirements, but two interesting ones come to mind.

Cyanide would work. It is extremely deadly, but in small doses may only make your reporter ill. A very small amount of either sodium or potassium cyanide, both white powders, could be sprinkled into the tobacco, and when smoked would be inhaled into the lungs. It is then rapidly absorbed into the bloodstream, and begins poisoning all the cells of the body.

The victim would become dizzy, short of breath, and may have chest pain, loss of consciousness, or seizures, and may die. If the dose was large, and if he smoked the entire cigarette, he could die in minutes. But if he only took a couple of drags, his exposure could be very light, only making him ill.

Another choice could be benzene. Benzene is a slightly sweet-smelling liquid that is used as a solvent in paints, oils, plastics, rubber, and many other products. It has a very low boiling point (the temperature at which it converts from a liquid to a gas), and is easily absorbed through the lungs.

If the cigarette had been treated with a small amount of liquid benzene, the heat of the burning tobacco would quickly convert it to a gas for inhalation. Symptoms onset immediately, and include weakness, dizziness, nausea, headache, chest pain, staggering, confusion, and loss of consciousness. Again, if exposure is high, death may occur.

Either of these could make your reporter ill. He would recover fairly quickly, but just might give up smoking. A win-win situation.

How Does "Sewer Gas" Kill?

Q: A terrorist organization is plotting to level a city by sabotaging the methane-stripping system in the local sewer. How long would it take for the gas to become explosive? What are the effects of sewer gas on a human being?

A: How long it would take for enough gas to accumulate so that a spark would cause an explosion would depend upon many factors, such as the size of the sewer system, the concentration of the methane, the rate at which it entered the area, and the degree of ventilation within the sewer. A civil engineer might be able help you with this, but since this is fiction, you can simply be vague about the exact time frame. An hour wouldn't likely be long enough, and a day or so would be more than sufficient.

"Sewer gas" is the term used to describe a combination of hydrogen sulfide, carbon monoxide (CO), and methane. It is occasionally responsible for the deaths of those who work in sewers and mines, areas where this gaseous combination tends to accumulate. Methane and CO kill by diminishing the percentage of the air that is oxygen, and this leads to asphyxiation. Hydrogen sulfide, a byproduct of the fermentation that often occurs in sewers and cesspools, is even more treacherous. When inhaled it combines with the blood's hemoglobin (the oxygen-carrying molecule found inside the red blood cells) and forms methemoglobin, a molecule that will not transport oxygen from the lungs to the body. This basically "suffocates" the body's cells. Methemoglobin imparts a dark purple color to the blood, and at autopsy the ME would find high levels of sulfide in the victim's blood.

Victims of sewer gas exposure develop progressive shortness of breath, cough, fatigue, weakness, confusion, disorientation, dizziness, poor coordination, a staggering gait, and finally coma and death. The treatment is to remove the victim from exposure and supply oxygen until the body rids itself of the sewer gas chemicals.

What Substance Added to a Massage Lotion Could Cause the Death of an Athlete?

Q: I have a character, a professional hockey player, who I would like to murder by way of a poison that is absorbed through the skin. I need something that can be placed in the lotion used for his pregame massage and that the trainer can wash off his own hands, avoiding self-poisoning. It also needs to take three to four hours to work. The idea is that the athlete has a massage prior to the game, plays a full game, and then is found dead either in a hot tub or on the massage table after the game is over. Is there such a substance, and if so, what would the symptoms be?

Terry Martens
Hamilton, Ontario, Canada

A: There aren't many toxins that absorb through the skin, and none would completely fit your requirements, mainly your timeline. Drugs that do pass through the skin and kill usually do so quickly, so it's the three- or four-hour delay that's the problem. But you might be able to work around this.

We can rule out several common poisons very quickly. Cyanide works in minutes and would also be absorbed through the hands of your trainer, so both the player and the trainer would be found dead in the training room. Heavy metals such as lead, mercury, and arsenic may also absorb through the skin, but they don't fit because, for the most part, each requires weeks of repetitive exposure to cause illness or death.

But topical sedatives such as fentanyl might work if you alter your timeline. As a sedative, fentanyl would make your hockey player very sleepy, and if enough were used could make him stop breathing, and die. Fentanyl comes in patches under the trade name Duragesic. This medication is used for pain relief in people with cancer and other diseases associated with severe pain. Other preparations are given by injection as a preop anesthetic. The Russians used an aerosolized version of fentanyl to subdue the Chechen rebels who took over a theater in Moscow a few years ago. It works very quickly when inhaled.

I would suggest that your hockey player have his massage after the game, which would make more sense anyway. Massage is to relax the muscles and help remove toxins such as lactic acid, and it is better done after exercise; before would be counterproductive. He could be the last person to get a postgame massage, and might doze off in the process, as the fentanyl takes effect. The masseuse might say, "I'm done," think the guy is going to wake up, and go shower, pack up his stuff, and leave, not realizing that the victim was actually slipping into a coma. After he left the guy would simply stop breathing and die. His teammates may have gone ahead to a local bar to celebrate, thinking he would show up later, and when he didn't someone could go look for him, and find him dead. The toxicologist might then find fentanyl in the massage oil or lotion and the investigation would go from there.

The only problem I see is that some of the drug would also absorb through the trainer's hands, so he might also begin to feel drowsy. But after a long day he might simply think he's tired. He might abbreviate the massage, go wash his hands, and then head home. Once the drug-laced lotion was washed away from his hands its effects would dissipate very quickly.

If My Killer Uses Abrin as His Poison of Choice, Will the ME Be Able to Find It?

Q: I want to write a story involving the use of abrin to kill a character. My dilemma is that I'm told that abrin cannot be traced during an autopsy; it can only be discovered through environmental observation. Is there a single test a shrewd ME can use to determine such a cause of death, or will the villain get away with this crime in my story?

A: Abrin is yellowish-white powder that is derived from the seeds of the rosary pea, also called the jequirity pea. These plants grow in many tropical areas of the world and, as with many toxic plants, it has been used in various herbal remedies over the years. The seeds, which are red with black on one end, are also used in making beaded jewelry, and an occasional poisoning occurs if the seeds are ingested. This is rare, so that any exposure to abrin is likely to be intentional.

Abrin is very stable and can be stored for many years. It can enter the body through ingestion, inhalation, and even by injection.

Abrin is similar to ricin, which comes from the castor bean, in that it is a metabolic poison. It enters the cells of the body and prevents them from manufacturing the proteins that they need to survive. The cells of the body then begin to die, and so does the victim. The symptoms that follow depend upon how it enters the body.

If eaten, the victim would develop symptoms as early as six hours later, but more likely wouldn't for one to three days. The symptoms would include nausea, vomiting, diarrhea (maybe bloody diarrhea), severe dehydration, shock, and death. He may also develop hallucinations, seizures, and bloody urine.

If inhaled, the symptoms begin within eight hours and include shortness of breath, cough, chest pain, nausea, and pulmonary edema (lungs full of water). The victim will literally drown in the water that collects within the lungs, suffer cardiac and respiratory failure, and die.

There is no known test for abrin, so the ME might not be able to determine the cause of death. That said, it might be possible for the ME to test some of the victim's stomach contents with gas chromatography and mass spectrometry—called GC/MS for short. The combination of these two techniques gives the chemical "fingerprint" of any substance. So if you want the drug found, have your ME and forensic toxicologist use GC/MS and come to the correct conclusion. If not, simply ignore this technique, since I know of no instance in which it has been used to find abrin. It's possible, though, so you can have it either way.

Could My Religious Terrorist Group Make Genetically Altered Toxic Corn?

Q: My dairy farmer protagonist feeds her cows with corn supplied to her by a neighbor. It turns out the corn has been genetically altered by a religious terrorist group. The corn does not affect the cows themselves, but rather the milk they produce. I realize this idea is rather far-fetched, but I'm hoping it is at least theoretically possible. The terrorists have added a fungal gene to the corn's DNA sequence, which in turn produces aflatoxin, a nasty biological poison.

My question is, what physical symptoms could I have the people show (keeping in mind that this is a far from realistic situation)? In my current draft the victims develop flulike symptoms, but I'm wondering if I should be more specific. Maybe vomiting, diarrhea, dehydration, and fever. Any suggestions?

Judy Clemens
Anthony- and Agatha-award-nominated author of the
Stella Crown series
www.judyclemens.com

A: You're correct. This is not a likely real-life scenario, but in fiction it is wonderfully wicked.

From a genetic point of view, the altering of the genetic sequence of the corn would be unlikely to affect the cow's milk and then in turn affect the child who consumed the milk. The digestive processes would likely denature the corn's DNA and proteins. This is true of most foodstuffs. Still, in fiction you could make a plausible case for this transfer occurring.

Aflatoxin can be harmless or, as you pointed out, a nasty toxin. It is a mycotoxin that is produced by certain types of *Aspergillus* fungi. *Aspergillus* itself can cause severe upper respiratory and lung infections that can be very difficult to treat, particularly in people with compromised immune systems.

The symptoms you outlined are what would be expected from an ingested toxin, so I think you are right on in that regard. Also, many of these fungal toxins can trigger allergic-type symptoms, such as itching, swelling of the face and hands, a skin rash, and asthma. Another GI symptom would be a malabsorption syndrome. If the toxin caused an allergic-type reaction within the intestines, the intestinal lining would become edematous (swollen with water) and inflamed. This would interfere with the absorption of nutrients, particularly fats and proteins. Malabsorption of fats would lead to bloating, abdominal cramps, gas, and perhaps oily, foul-smelling stools. Malabsorption of protein, if it continued for several weeks or months, would lead to fatigue, weight loss, and muscle wasting.

Another thing you might want to look at are prions. These are the presumptive causative agents in mad cow disease. They are abnormal proteins that pass from the ingested meat into the person's bloodstream, and then to the brain, where they work their mischief. They are extremely hardy and even survive cremation of the cow's remains. The ashes produced from an infected cow remain infectious, and are handled in a fashion similar to nuclear waste.

Obviously, you don't want your victims to get a disease like mad cow (a type of spongiform encephalitis), but again this is fiction.

You could create your own prion-mediated disease that wasn't uniformly fatal but rather made the victims very ill.

What Veterinary Medicine Could Be Used to Kill One of My Characters?

Q: I'm a mystery writer working on a story set in horse country. My bad guy has access to many types of veterinary medications, and he plans to use one of them to do away with an elderly person. He is counting on no autopsy being performed. My question is, what medication could my villain use that is not detectable at autopsy?

G. M. Malliet

www.publishersmarketplace.com/members/gmalli/

A: One of the most common animal tranquilizers is PCP, or phencyclidine. It is also a common drug of abuse, so your perpetrator could get it from a vet's office, a horse farm, or on the street. It goes by the slang names angel dust, crystal, hog, tic, zoot, and others. It can be swallowed, snorted, or smoked, and is often sprinkled on a marijuana joint.

PCP is what is called a dissociative anesthetic. This means that it not only sedates but also causes a dissociative psychiatric reaction, which is a partial or complete loss of contact with reality. It often mimics acute paranoid schizophrenia. This is one of the things that make it dangerous. The user loses the ability to understand his situation and will often do foolhardy things, such as walk into traffic or try to fly out a window.

Its effects on a given individual are unpredictable, but besides a dissociation reaction it can cause euphoria; delusional thinking; hallucinations (mostly auditory and visual); feelings of distorted time and space, or of floating or weightlessness; poor concentration; anxiety; panic; paranoia; aggressive and violent behavior; loss of pain sense; nausea; vomiting; high blood pressure; sweating; rapid heart beat; very high or very low body temperatures;

seizures; coma; brain hemorrhage; muscle damage; and other pleasant things.

Your perpetrator could slip some into the victim's food or drink, or inject him with a bit and let the drug do its work. If swallowed the effects would begin in fifteen minutes or so. If injected or smoked or snorted the effects would be immediate. Your victim could then get in a car and drive into a tree or off a cliff. Since his contact with reality would be impaired he might believe he's a fighter pilot or playing a video game. Or your victim could develop any and all of the above symptoms and die.

There are no visible signs at autopsy of PCP intoxication, but it might be found with a drug screen. If the ME wrote off the death to an accident or a natural death from a cardiac arrhythmia, no one would know that your villain had done him in. But even if the PCP were found, the death could still be deemed accidental if the ME believed that the victim had taken the drug himself for recreational reasons. Not likely in an elderly person, but anything is possible.

Can Botox Be Used as a Weapon for Murder?

Q: Is it possible for my antagonist to kill someone with Botox?

Jennifer Apodaca
Author of *Thrilled to Death* and other Samantha Shaw
mysteries
www.jenniferapodaca.com

A: The short answer is yes. Botox is a commercial preparation of the botulinum toxin, which is produced by the bacterium *Clostridium botulinum*. Actually, this organism produces seven types of botulinum toxin. Botox contains small doses of botulinum A, and when used appropriately is safe. The problem arises if too much is given, or if one of the many knockoff versions, which are brought into the country illegally, are used. These non–FDA–approved versions might contain larger amounts of the toxin.

Botulinum toxin is a neurotoxin (affects the nerves or the area where the nerves attach to the muscles) that leads to flaccid (limp) muscular paralysis. This means that the muscles relax and cannot contract. When injected into the forehead the muscles in the area are paralyzed, become lax, and wrinkles disappear. So far so good. But if too much is given, the toxin can enter the bloodstream, travel throughout the body, and paralyze all the muscles, including those needed for respiration. The person can then die from asphyxia. This is an unlikely occurrence, but can happen.

So giving someone a large dose of botulinum toxin can cause death. How much? It depends upon many things, including the age, weight, and general health of the victim, as well as the actual concentration of the toxin in the preparation used. For your story, don't get caught up in the details, but rather simply fill a syringe with the drug and inject it.

What Toxin Could Be Used in a "Frozen Bullet" and Bring About the Sudden Death of My Victim?

Q: In my story a professional assassin kills a U.S. senator. I thought about having her shoot him, but I want the cause of his death to be more mysterious. My plan is to have her use a liquid poison that she freezes into a bullet and fires from a rifle at a safe distance. The frozen bullet would dissolve into a packet of liquid by the time it reaches him, so that no entry wound would occur. My question is, what liquid toxin would kill him instantly?

Kathleen Antrim
Author of *Capital Offense*
www.kathleenantrim.com

A: I love your method of doing in the unfortunate senator. A frozen bullet is both ingenious and unexpected, and the use of a toxin makes it even better. Not the cliché icicle knife that leaves a wound but no weapon.

Obviously your killer will have to calculate at what temperature to freeze the bullet and how far it must travel before liquefying. The result would be that the bullet reaches the victim as a high-speed liquid packet not unlike the needleless injectors used for immunizations today. In these the column of liquid medicine is fired at high speed into the skin. It leaves behind only a small mark, less than a metallic needle. It is likely that the unfortunate senator would have a bruise or small abrasion at the point of impact, but this might be deemed of no concern by the coroner. After all, who would consider a liquid bullet?

So your chosen method of delivery is cool and clever, to say the least. But what toxin would fit the bill? Sodium azide.

Sodium azide is a liquid that is highly toxic and absorbs rapidly through the skin, so breakage of the skin is not necessary. It has several catastrophic effects that could lead to a quick death. It causes a rapid and significant drop in blood pressure, leading to shock and death. It is also what we call a "metabolic poison" in that it shuts down the inner workings of the body's cells and results in rapid death.

The combination of this sudden drop in blood pressure and the poisoning of cells would lead to a sudden collapse, and it would look very much like a heart attack to any observer. There would be no wound and no abnormalities found on autopsy, so the ME might write the death off to a deadly cardiac arrhythmia. Toxicological testing would show nothing unless the ME specifically tested for sodium azide, and he'd most likely never consider that.

Can Death from an Injection of Methylene Chloride Be Disguised to Look Like a Death from Carbon Monoxide Inhalation?

Q: I have two murders committed by altering a car and a furnace to emit carbon monoxide. For the third murder in my story I want to inject the already-sedated victim with something and still have the death be due to carbon monoxide. I understand that inhaling the fumes of methylene chloride causes the liver to give off carbon monoxide, which then forms carboxyhemoglobin in the blood, as would carbon monoxide inhalation. Would an injection of methylene chloride do the same, and if so what amount would need to be given?

A: Methylene chloride, also called dichloromethane, is a colorless liquid with an astringent yet slightly sweet odor, similar to ether. And like ether it is volatile, which means it readily evaporates into a gas. It is made from methane or methanol (wood or denatured alcohol), and is found in paint thinners and strippers and some metal degreasers, as well as in some pesticides. Most industrial and accidental exposures are from inhalation or skin contact.

Contact can cause burning and irritation of the skin and eyes. Inhalation may cause similar burning of the bronchi (breathing tubes), with coughing and shortness of breath. Dizziness, nausea, vomiting, headache, confusion, giddiness, disorientation, and numbness and tingling of the extremities may follow. Ingestion can produce all the above symptoms, as well as burning and irritation of the mouth, esophagus, and stomach.

As it is broken down in the body it is converted to formic acid, which is excreted through the kidneys, and carbon monoxide (CO), which attaches to the hemoglobin of the blood, producing carboxyhemoglobin. Since this replaces oxyhemoglobin (the oxygen-hemoglobin complex that carries oxygen from the lungs to the tissues), the victim is basically starved for oxygen, and this results in many of the above symptoms and may cause death, particularly in persons with heart or lung disease.

I could find no information on the injection of this compound, probably because you're the only one diabolical enough to consider it. But let's look at what might happen based on the properties of the compound. First of all, it would burn severely when injected. If your victim is heavily sedated, this may not be a problem for your killer. Since it is very volatile it may also form tiny gas bubbles of methylene chloride in the body, and these could go to the heart and kill the victim fairly quickly. If not, the liver would go to work on it and would convert it to formic acid and CO, just as it would if it had been absorbed through the lungs or stomach.

The CO levels could rise rapidly, and thus the carboxyhemoglobin level, and your character would not likely be long for this world. How much? I have no way of knowing, so I would suggest simply glossing over it in your story. I'd have the perpetrator give the victim a full syringe.

The ME would have little problem determining the elevated carboxyhemoglobin in the victim's blood. And that might be as far as he goes. If the victim was found in a CO-rich environment, that is. You would need to stage this murder to look like one of the others you mentioned. Finding evidence of CO intoxication in someone who wasn't exposed to CO would raise a few eyebrows and cause a more thorough search to be launched. But if the victim were found in his garage with his car engine running, the ME would have no reason to suspect that something else was involved.

Or he could find the needle mark or discover that the victim's blood is very acidic. Further toxicological testing might then reveal the formic acid and the methylene chloride in the victim. A murder investigation would follow.

Either way works.

How Does the Toxin of the Poisonous California Newt Bring About Death?

Q: I want to use an unusual poison in my story. If you milked the toxin from the skin of a California newt, or perhaps from poisonous frogs found in a university research lab, and applied it to chocolate candies, would it kill a person? Would one treated chocolate be enough? What would the symptoms be, and how long would it take to die?

Barbara A. Herdman
Urbana, Missouri

A: California newts (*Taricha torosa*) are large salamanders that grow to be up to eight inches in length. They live along the coastal areas of California. They are reddish-brown on top and have a yellow-orange belly. Their toxin is called tarichatoxin, which is similar to tetrodotoxin found in the puffer fish. It is a neurotoxin in that it blocks nerve transmission and causes muscular paralysis and death from asphyxia when the victim's breathing ceases.

But by using frogs from a research lab you open up another entire world of possibilities, frogs that are much more toxic than the newt. Each of these also produces powerful neurotoxins and causes death by paralysis and asphyxia.

Dart frogs of the genus *Phyllobates* are very toxic. They come from tropical rain forests in Brazil and other areas in South America. Most are brightly colored and secrete a toxin from their skin. Natives use their toxin to "poison" their darts to tranquilize prey.

The golden-colored *Phyllobates terribilis* contains the toxin batrachotoxin, which it secretes from skin glands. Since this toxin is deadly to other animals, it makes an excellent deterrent against getting eaten. It is very potent, and only a very small amount—maybe the size of a couple of grains of sand—is all that is needed to bring about death.

Another poisonous genus is termed the *Dendrobates. Dendrobates tinctorius*, a small frog with a black-and-white body and blue legs, and the beautiful *Dendrobates azureus*, the blue dart frog, which is several shades of blue, produce the toxin pumiliotoxin. This toxin is similar to but less powerful than batrachotoxin but can still be very deadly.

There are, of course, many others.

Each of these toxins is very potent, and only a very small amount would be needed. For your scenario a few drops of the toxin placed in or on a chocolate could be very deadly very quickly. The symptoms would begin about fifteen minutes or so after ingestion, with weakness, shortness of breath, and a numb feeling. This would progress over the next fifteen minutes or so, until the victim collapsed, stopped breathing, and died.

What Substance Can My Soft-Hearted Thief Use to Sedate the Dogs That Guard the Estates He Robs?

Q: In the novel I am writing, a thief with a tender heart breaks into estates to rob those who are stealing from the poor and middle class. However, he does not want to kill guard dogs when they are present. What can he mix into some raw hamburger that will put them to sleep in a short time, keep them under for about two hours, and allow them to wake with no negative after effects?

> Lucy Kaufman (writing as Lucy Simons)
> Author of *Soul Food: Feeding the Inner Spirit* and *Killing Grandma and Other Family Issues*

A: There are several possibilities.

Acepromazine, sold as PromAce Rx, is a veterinary drug that is very effective. It comes in 25-mg tablets, and can be found in a vet office. The dose for sedating a dog is .25 to 1.0 mgs per pound of body weight. For a 50- to 60-pound guard dog 2 to 3 tablets would do the trick. It might take 30 minutes to work, but if you doubled the dose (5 or 6 tablets), it could take as little as 15 minutes.

Valium (diazepam) is common and widely available. Many people have this in their medicine cabinets. The effective dosage is about 2 mgs per kg. One kg equals 2.2 pounds. This means that the dose is roughly 1 mg per pound. For a 50-pound dog, 10 5-mg Valium tablets could be crushed and mixed with meat. It might take 15 to 30 minutes to work.

Xanax (alprazolam) is also common and readily available. Like Valium, this is found in many medicine cabinets. The dose here would be 0.1 mg per kg. For the same dog as above your thief would need about 2.5 to 3 mgs for sedation. Xanax comes in 0.25- and 0.5-mg tablets. If you crushed six 0.5 mg tablets, it should be enough. Count on 15 to 30 minutes for full effect.

What Happens When Someone Is Poisoned Slowly with Selenium?

Q: I'm about to start my next novel, which will involve a chronic poisoning over a period of time. I'm looking for a substance that would cause death disguised as natural illness. I thought of arsenic but feel it is too commonplace. I saw a TV play based on a true story about a man who was murdering his wife with selenium in her shampoo. The doctors couldn't figure out what was making her sick. Is this a good method, or can you suggest other poisons that would have that effect, and describe the symptoms they would cause?

> Patricia Harwin
> Author of *Arson and Old Lace* and *Slaying Is Such Sweet Sorrow*

A: Selenium is a nonmetallic element in the same chemical family as sulfur, oxygen, polonium, and tellurium. It is an element essential for life, and deficiency can lead to various medical problems, the most important being cardiomyopathy (a weakening of the heart muscle). Interestingly, Marco Polo may have discovered the first cases of selenium poisoning when he described a disease called "hoof rot," which occurred in horses in the Nan Shan and Tien Shan mountains of southern China. The soil in that area is rich in selenium.

Selenium poisoning is rare, though it does occur in industrial situations. Its principal applications are in the manufacture of glass, ceramics, photoelectric cells, semiconductors, steel, and vulcanized rubber. The most toxic forms are selenium dioxide (SeO_2) and selenious acid (H_2SeO_4).

Acute poisoning is most often lethal. The ingestion or inhalation of selenium dioxide or selenious acid (found in gun bluing solutions) can cause a dramatic drop in blood pressure due to its toxic effects on the heart muscle and a dilation (opening up) of the blood vessels throughout the body. These effects can lead to cardiac arrest and death. It can also cause severe burns to the skin and the lining of the mouth, as well as the lungs, where bleeding and pulmonary edema (lungs filled with water) may result. A reddish pigmentation of the teeth, hair, and nails, coupled with a garliclike odor to the breath, are typical of acute poisoning.

Chronic poisoning occurs with long-term, low-level exposure. The victim's skin may develop a reddish hue, and a pruritic (itchy) scalp rash may appear. The hair becomes brittle and breaks easily or falls out. The nails become brittle and display red or yellowish-white transverse or longitudinal lines. The breath smells of garlic, and the victim may complain of a metallic taste in the mouth. Nausea, vomiting, fatigue, irritability, labile emotions, depression, tremors, and muscle tenderness may also occur.

The diagnosis of selenium poisoning, either in the living or at autopsy, is made by testing the victim's blood and urine for increased selenium levels. At autopsy, findings would likely include congestion in the lungs and kidneys, patchy scarring and enlargement of the heart, edema and swelling of the brain, and an orange-brown discoloration of the skin and internal organs.

Treatment for those who survive the exposure consists of stopping the chronic exposure and using intramuscular doses of dimercaprol (BAL, or British Anti-Lewisite), which acts as a chelating agent by binding the selenium and removing it from the body through the kidneys. The usual schedule is to inject 3 to 5 mgs per kg of body weight every 4 hours for 2 days, every 6 hours on the third day, and then every 12 hours thereafter for 10 days.

For your purposes, either an acute or chronic poisoning could work, depending upon whether you want the person to die right away or slowly, over a month or so. Gun bluing solutions contain lethal amounts of selenious acid. A couple of tablespoons added to food or drink could kill the person in a couple of hours. Adding a little here and a little there day by day would accomplish a chronic poisoning. The victim would gradually become sicker. Her appetite would disappear, her weight would drop, and nausea and vomiting would occur. Her hair would fall out, and she would become weak and short of breath. She would become irritable, and her hands would develop a tremor. She might develop heart failure and pulmonary edema. If she visited her M.D., the doctor might diagnose heart disease or gastroenteritis, even the flu. Selenium poisoning would never enter his mind. As the condition progressed she might be hospitalized, where she could die of progressive heart failure. Since this is a common occurrence, the death would likely be written off as heart disease. That is, until your protagonist became suspicious and tracked down the true cause of the victim's demise.

Can the Abortive Herb Tansy Cause Death?

Q: A central character in my story, which is set in Oklahoma in 1909, is a progressively and severely depressed woman, a mother of three in a dysfunctional marriage, who is unwillingly impregnated for a fourth time. She determines to abort the child, and enlists the aid of a woman who grows tansy, which I understand was one of the preferred methods of abortion at that time. I believe it can also be deadly, which is the result in my story.

Exactly what happens when the tansy tea is drunk? Would it provoke vomiting, cramps, hemorrhaging? In what time frame would these things happen? I need to set the stage for when a doctor is called in later to verify a death from what he is told have been "rather bad intestinal episodes."

Trudy Graham
Tulsa, Oklahoma
Author of *Godforsaken* and *Dear God, What Do I Do Now?*

A: Tansy (*Tanacetum vulgare*), also called bachelor's button, is a fernlike plant with yellow flowers. It grows throughout Europe and in the eastern and Pacific Northwest regions of the United States. The leaves, flowers, stems, and seeds contain the toxic oil tenacetin, which is the active ingredient.

It has been used as an herbal medicine for centuries, and was apparently used in certain "witchcraft rituals" in the Middle Ages. Physicians and herbalists recommended it for the treatment of intestinal worms, gout, skin rashes, arthritis, sprains, and wounds; as a bitter stimulant and tonic; to relieve intestinal spasms and gas; and as an emmenagogue—to promote the onset of menses. It is this last effect that made it an effective abortive.

Traditionally it has been prepared as a powder by grinding the leaves, as an oil by pressing the leaves and collecting the extract, or as a tea by steeping the leaves in hot water. The roots were often mixed with sugar or honey for the treatment of gout.

The toxic symptoms of tansy ingestion begin an hour or more after intake. They include salivation, nausea, vomiting, dilated (enlarged) pupils, rapid pulse, abdominal cramping, vaginal bleeding, seizures, and death. These can occur in any degree and in any combination, depending upon the dose and the particular person's response to the drug.

Your character could drink some of the tea, and an hour or so later begin to develop nausea and abdominal cramping, with or without vomiting. She would then begin to experience vaginal bleeding, and would abort the fetus. This would likely take two to three hours after ingestion, but the range is quite broad, so you can make it anywhere from two to eight hours as needed for your plot. She could then experience seizures (or not—up to you) and die. The physician wouldn't likely suspect tansy, and would consider the death due to an intestinal ailment or a miscarriage. Death from either of these was not uncommon in 1909.

Part III

The Police, the Crime Scene, and the Crime Lab

When Can the Police Move a Corpse at a Crime Scene?

Q: I have the police showing up at a suspect's house to find him shot in the head and lying on the floor, facedown. When is it okay for them to turn over the body? Once pictures have been taken?

A: They wouldn't. At least, they shouldn't.

The first officer on the scene should quickly and as unobtrusively as possible make sure the victim is indeed dead. If not, he should activate the EMS system immediately. If so, he should secure the scene and touch nothing until the detectives, CSI personnel, and coroner's technicians arrive. At a crime scene the scene itself belongs to the police, but the body belongs to the coroner or ME. Only the coroner's tech should examine, roll, move, wrap, or transport the body.

Yes, the entire scene, as well as selective close-up shots (wounds, evidence, blood spatters, footprints, etc.), would be photographed before anything is touched or moved.

At least, that's the way it should work. Doesn't mean it always does. So your cops could do almost anything you wanted them to do. And their actions might contaminate, render unusable, or cause a judge to toss out any of the evidence.

How Long Does It Take Blood to Clot When Spilled on a Tile Floor?

Q: In my story a murder is committed by a violent slashing across either the carotid or jugular vessels in the victim's

neck. How long would it take the blood, if spilled on a
tile floor, to coagulate?

A: The type of injury you describe would produce rapid loss of
blood if either vessel were severed. With the jugular vein the blood
would be dark purple (venous blood is purple because it is poor in
oxygen), and it would gush out and flow over the victim or the
floor or whatever was downhill from the laceration site. As the victim bled out, the flow of blood would slow to a trickle, and ultimately stop. If the carotid artery were slashed, the bleeding would
be arterial. That is, it would exit the wound in long, pulsing, bright
red squirts (arterial blood is red because it is rich in oxygen) that
could travel several feet. The arch-shaped or cascadelike pattern
these pulses would leave on a wall, floor, or anywhere they struck is
called an arterial spatter pattern. The spurts would weaken, and
these arching spatters would become smaller as the victim lost
blood volume and his blood pressure dropped. As the victim slipped
into shock and neared death, the bleeding would finally slow to a
trickle, and stop.

Regardless of how blood leaves the body it will clot in about
five to fifteen minutes, and will be dark maroon, gelatinlike, and
sticky to the touch. Over a couple of hours it will separate into a
dark maroon or blackish clot surrounded by a pale yellow serum.
This is due to some contraction of the clotted blood and a
"squeezing out" of the serum, which is not involved in the clotting
process.

We do this in the lab quite often, since many blood tests are
done on the serum and not on whole blood. The blood is allowed
to clot in a test tube and the tube is placed into a centrifuge and
spun rapidly for several minutes. This pushes the clotted blood into
the bottom of the tube and the clear, yellow serum floats on top.
The serum is then removed and used for various tests.

The blood on the floor will dry to a crusty brownish state over
twelve hours or up to three or four days, depending upon the
amount of blood present, the ambient temperature, the humidity
level, and the degree of ventilation. A small amount will dry faster
than a large collection, and warmer, drier, and breezy conditions

would dry any amount faster than conditions that are cool, damp, and still.

How Exactly Does a Corpse Decay, and What Makes a Body Float When Disposed of in a Body of Water?

Q: My homicide detective finds a corpse floating in the San Francisco Bay. I need to know what actually happens when a body decays, what makes it a floater, and what a corpse in water for several weeks would look like.

A: Under normal circumstances, the decomposition of a body follows a predictable pattern, which the ME can use in his estimation of the time of death. Decomposition actually involves two distinct processes: autolysis and putrefaction.

Autolysis is basically a process of self-digestion. After death the enzymes within the body's cells begin the chemical breakdown of the tissues. As with most chemical reactions the process is hastened by heat and slowed by cold.

Putrefaction is the bacteria-mediated destruction of the body's tissues. The bacteria responsible come mostly from the intestinal tract of the deceased, though environmental bacteria and yeasts contribute in many situations. Bacteria thrive in warm, moist environments and become sluggish in colder climes. Freezing will stop their activities completely. A frozen body will not undergo putrefaction until it thaws.

Putrefaction is an ugly and unpleasant process, and under normal temperate conditions follows a known sequence. During the first twenty-four hours the abdomen takes on a greenish discoloration, which spreads to the neck, shoulders, and head. Bloating follows. This is due to the accumulation of gas, a by-product of the actions of the bacteria within the body's cavities and skin. Swelling begins in the face, where the features expand and the eyes and tongue protrude. The skin will then begin to "marble." This is a weblike patterning of the blood vessels over the face, chest, abdomen, and extremities. The pattern is green-black in color, and is due to the reaction of the blood's hemoglobin with hydrogen sulfide, a chemical produced by the decay process. As gases continue to accumulate, the abdomen swells and the skin begins to blister. Soon skin and hair slippage occur, and the fingernails begin to slough off. By this stage the body has taken on a greenish-black color, and the fluids of decomposition (purge fluids) begin to drain from the nose and mouth. This may look like bleeding from trauma, but it is due to the extensive breakdown of the body's tissues.

The rate at which this process occurs is almost never normal because the conditions surrounding the body are almost never normal. Both environmental and internal body conditions alter this process greatly. Obesity, excess clothing, a hot and humid environment, and the presence of sepsis (an infection in the bloodstream) may speed this process, so that its condition within twenty-four hours appears like five or six days have passed. On the other hand, a thin, unclothed corpse lying on a cold surface with a cool breeze would follow a much slower decomposition process. Very cold climes may slow the process so much that even after several months the body appears as if it has been dead only a day or two. Freezing will protect the body from putrefaction if the body is frozen before the process begins. Once putrefaction sets in, even freezing the body may not prevent its eventual decay. If frozen quickly enough, the body may be preserved for years.

Now let's look at floaters. "Floaters" is the term used to describe corpses found floating in water. When tossed into a lake, bay, or other body of water, corpses initially sink. But as the gas by-products of decay collect within the tissues and the abdomen, the corpse will become buoyant and float to the surface. How long does this take? The rate of this gas accumulation is directly related to the ambient temperature. Warmer water increases bacterial growth, hastens the decay process, and causes a more rapid accumulation of gas. In very warm water, such as a Florida swamp in August, this might take only a couple of days. In cold water, such as the San Francisco Bay, this may take several months. The general rule is that one week on land equals two weeks in the water, assuming the temperature is the same. Your corpse would be in very cold water, so it might not pop up for two to four weeks, maybe even a bit longer, and might look more like a week-old corpse (perhaps with a bit more swelling and softening of the skin, due to prolonged water submersion, and maybe some evidence of damage by marine creatures).

How Long Will Evidence Survive on a Corpse or a Murder Weapon That Is in Water?

Q: My question is in regards to the forensic evidence that can be collected from a body or a murder weapon that is found in a river or washed up on the beach. How much evidence does water actually wash away? The scenario is that a person is knifed to death, the body and murder weapon dumped in a nearby lake, or river, or off a pier (hopefully it doesn't matter). Will the bloodstains on the victim's garments be washed off? What about fibers and hair samples and DNA evidence? Would it wash away fingerprints from the murder weapon or the body? What evidence can, in fact, be collected? And does the time in which the body is found make a difference? Finding the body the next day as opposed to a few weeks later?

C. Cicchini
Sydney, Australia

A: The bottom line is that whatever happens, happens. All of the evidence could be washed away, or some if it, or none of it. Anything is possible. Blood, hair, fibers could be found or not. The most important factors would be the activity of the water and the length of time the corpse or weapon was in the water. If the body were in a quiet pond, still lake, or in a protected area along a river where the flow of water is minimal, more evidence would be left, and it would survive for a longer period of time, maybe days or weeks. If the corpse was in a rapidly flowing river, tumbling down the river, or in ocean waves, then all the evidence could be washed away in a matter of minutes. And anything in between.

These are general rules. A body could tumble a mile down a river, over a waterfall, and be trapped by a tree limb in the path of the moving water and still have blood, hair, and fibers present when examined. And a body in a calm pond could have none. It's extremely variable. I know of one case where a rape-murder victim was tossed in a river and pulled out five hours later. Enough saliva was found in a bite mark on her shoulder to get DNA that matched the suspect. So anything is possible.

Even if all the visible blood was leeched from the victim's clothing, there still may be enough soaked into the materials that blood typing and DNA matching is possible. Also, blood may collect in the groove between the knife blade and handle, and it may survive the water exposure. Hairs and fibers may become entangled in the victim's hair or clothing and be found. Fingerprints may survive on the weapon but not on the body. Fingerprints are very rarely found on skin, and, in general, only last about ninety minutes on the living and up to twenty-four hours on a corpse. Add to this the effects of moving water, and finding prints would be very unlikely, even if the body were found quickly.

All this uncertainty is good, since you can craft your story any way you wish and it will work.

Can the Fingerprint of a Perpetrator Be Lifted from the Victim's Severed Finger?

Q: Is it possible to lift a suspect's fingerprint from a victim's severed finger? In my story the bad guys send a severed finger along with a ransom note. They are careful not to touch the ransom note, envelope, or box, but could there be a print remaining on the cut-off finger? Maybe the fingernail?

Philip S. Donlay
Author of *Category Five* and *Code Black*
www.philipdonlay.com

A: Rarely prints can be lifted from human flesh, but not very often. They may remain on the skin of the living for up to ninety minutes, and on a corpse for up to twenty-four hours. And this is under perfect conditions. Finding prints on a severed finger would be extremely unlikely. Could it be found on the nail? Maybe. It would last longer there, and if the nail was polished or, better yet, had acrylic nails, the substrate might be hard enough to hold the print.

If the victim is a woman, she could have recently painted her nails, and they could still be slightly tacky. Touching them could leave behind a three-dimensional print. These are called plastic prints. It is like touching paint that hasn't completely dried. If the polish then dried and hardened, the print could be very well preserved.

Can Fingerprints Be Obtained from a Plastic Bag?

Q: Can fingerprints be found on a plastic bag like the ones you see in supermarkets? Also, does a person leave useful traces of himself in a pair of leather or woolen gloves?

Mat Coward
Author of *Open & Closed* and *Over & Under*
hometown.aol.co.uk/matcoward

A: Maybe, maybe not. It depends. A fingerprint results when oils and dirt from the finger are deposited on another surface. If a good print is left on a plastic bag or sheet, and if the plastic is in a relatively protected area so that the print is preserved until the bag is found, then it is often possible to find the print. Several methods will be employed.

Often using an angled or colored light will reveal the print. Certain laser lights and ultraviolet (UV) light may cause the oils in the print to fluoresce (glow slightly), and thus reveal the print. Colored and/or magnetic powders may show them too. Fuming with iodine and superglue (cyanoacrylate) may also expose these latent prints.

The bottom line is that prints can be lifted from plastic materials if the conditions are right. More than one case has been solved by such findings. I remember one where the print was found on the inside surface of a latex surgical-type glove that the perpetrator had worn to prevent leaving prints but then foolishly discarded, in a place they could be found.

Yes, the perpetrator could leave behind valuable evidence in a leather or woolen glove. His hair, the hair of his pet, and fibers from his clothes, car, or home could be deposited on or in the glove. If he bled or sweated on or in the glove, DNA might be found. Paint, mud, oils, plant materials, and other substances found on the glove might be traced back to his home or business. This is why the perfect crime is an illusion. It's the little and unexpected things that all too often trip up even the cleverest criminal.

How Long Will a Corpse Bleed After Death?

Q: A character in my story dies from jagged cuts to the throat. The body lies on its side. It's a hot, humid day. How long will blood trickle from the wound after death?

Judy Creekmore
LaPlace, Louisiana

A: Dead folks don't bleed. They may trickle and ooze for a few minutes, but they won't bleed. The reason is that blood flow ceases at death. When the heart stops beating, blood flow halts immediately, so blood no longer enters a wound. And if there is no blood, there is no bleeding. Any blood loss that does occur after death is oozing and trickling. This would follow the law of gravity, so only wounds on the downside of the body would ooze.

Your victim's wounds will, of course, bleed as long as his heart is beating, but will halt at death. I assume you're asking how much more bleeding will occur after that time. For your victim, he would need to fall facedown or on the side where the wound occurred for any significant oozing to occur. If the left side of your victim's neck is slashed, and he fell on his left side, gravity would allow some blood to continue seeping from the wound and onto the floor. Wounds on the upside of the body would not ooze, since that would be against gravity. Regardless, the blood would clot in five to fifteen minutes, and all oozing and trickling would stop. The hot humid day would have little effect on this.

Most of the blood found at the crime scene would have exited the victim's body while he was still alive. Very little would be from the slow oozing. But the pattern of the blood may tell a story. A large amount of pooled blood around the victim's head would suggest that the jugular vein might have been cut, while spurtlike stains might indicate that the carotid artery had been severed. The ME can use this to reconstruct the crime scene, and then use this information to test the credibility of any witnesses or suspects.

How Would the Police Examine the Car of a Man Who Has Disappeared?

Q: I'm hoping you can help me with a question for my current crime novel. A man has disappeared. The police find his abandoned car in a car park, with no signs of a struggle within. When they take the car away for examining, what would they be looking for? What examination would be performed on the inside of the car?

A: In short, they would look for anything and everything. The only limitations would be the aggressiveness (or lack thereof) of the investigators and the budget they had to work within.

They would impound the car and treat it as a crime scene even though they would not necessarily have evidence that a crime had occurred. Your character may simply have run off, or he may have been abducted or murdered. Their initial thoughts would be guided to some extent by where, when, and in what condition the car was found. For example, a car found in a lake would bring up different possibilities than one found in an airport parking lot.

They would remove every item from the car, place it in an evidence bag, and examine it at the crime lab for everything from prints to body fluids to trace evidence (hair, fibers, and the like). Everything from a wallet to a gun to a McDonald's wrapper.

They would dust the car inside and out for fingerprints, and would take samples of any fluids or stains in the car or the trunk to test for blood and other body fluids. They would vacuum the car for trace evidence and analyze any such evidence, and they might use Luminol to expose any invisible bloodstains. Any blood, tissue, or other evidence found would be carefully analyzed and stored.

They would keep the car impounded until the case was resolved or until no further evidence could be gleaned.

Can Illegally Manufactured Drugs Be Traced to a Common Source?

Q: If the police confiscate drugs in two different busts, can the lab determine that they came from the same batch? What types of tests are performed to uncover this connection?

A: The answer is probably yes, maybe no. Which means that in your story you can have it either way.

When any illicit drug is made—heroin, Ecstasy, whatever—each batch differs slightly in the types and amounts of the impurities that are always present. The maker never measures the ingredients absolutely accurately and never repeats the process exactly the same way. It's like your mother's cooking. She knows how to do it and just does it without sweating the minutiae. Drug cooks do the same thing. This may be useful in matching a drug sample to a specific cook or to a specific batch.

For example, one drug maker may use one type of talc as a cutting agent and another may use a different one. And each of them would use different amounts of talc in different batches. This means that the batches would vary not only in the amounts of talc but also in the exact chemical makeup of the talc used.

The most individualizing test for any chemical compound or mixture of compounds is the combination of gas chromatography and mass spectrometry (GC/MS). GC separates a mixture into its component compounds and MS gives the exact and completely individual "chemical fingerprint" of each of the compounds. It is highly specific and accurate.

Using GC/MS one can dissect any compound or mixture of compounds to an incredibly accurate degree, and can thus determine that the drugs came from different batches and/or from different manufacturers.

This same testing can often separate gasoline by manufacturer, batch, and sometimes even by the station where it was purchased. This can be critical to solving a case of arson. The same principle applies to clandestine drug labs.

If a Field Containing Several Corpses Is Discovered, How Would the Bodies Be Removed for Examination?

Q: In my story a construction crew digging up an old football field finds a skeleton. Then three more, and the FBI is called in. They arrive with their evidence response unit and start what is basically an archeological dig. Is that right? What I need are some specific things as to what this crew would do. The bodies are all two to three feet under the ground, and are strapped to and posed on some steel rebar. There will eventually be thirty-one bodies. How would the search team go about locating and digging up the bodies?

> Paul Guyot
> St. Louis, Missouri
> paulguyot.net

A: The search would follow a very organized pattern. The area would be laid out in a grid, usually by using stakes and string to form a pattern over the area to be searched. These grids may be any size, but 10 to 20 feet square would be about right. If the entire field is to be searched the grids might be a bit larger. This is all up to the officer in charge of the search. Teams of one or two would search for the bodies square by square in an inside-out, outside-in, or back-and-forth pattern.

There are several techniques for locating buried corpses, but since your killer has attached his victims to metal rebar, there is one very easy method—metal detectors. They would carefully sweep each grid and mark the locations of any metal found. Digging would then begin.

Perhaps some bodies will not be strapped to rebar so there is no metal to detect. Metal detectors may still be useful in locating victims' watches, jewelry, belt buckles, and other metallic materials. To find corpses that have absolutely no metal they might employ cadaver dogs or ground-penetrating radar. Both of these work better with a true corpse than with a skeleton, but these techniques might still work. The dogs smell and point on decaying flesh, so the presence of decaying tissue is important. They might even scent on skeletal remains. The radar depends upon changes in the reflected signal that occurs with a buried corpse. The reflection pattern reveals an object, and the officers must then dig it up to determine what it is. Again, an intact corpse is easier than a skeleton to see on the radar. This device is like a large shoebox with a long handle, and the user passes it over the area of search until he sees something on the screen.

Once the bodies have been located each will be excavated in an archeological fashion. The goal is to locate, gather, and preserve each piece of evidence (bones, jewelry, clothing, bullets, whatever is present) without missing, losing, or damaging it. Digging will be done carefully, and all the surrounding soil will be painstakingly searched and sifted. This might reveal teeth or bullets or rings, or many other small items of evidence.

The searchers would wear latex surgical-type gloves and use brushes, tweezers, ice pick–like probes (to move things around), magnifying glasses, and a square wooden or plastic box with a screen bottom for sifting the soil.

They might also employ ultraviolet (UV) light (black light) to look for bone fragments and hair and fibers. Bone tends to have a faint pale bluish ghostly glow under UV light. They might also slip on goggles and use various laser lights to scan the area. Different materials—such as cloth fibers and hair—may pop out under various laser lights when viewed through lenses of various types and colors of glass. Lumped together all these various types of lights are called alternative light sources, or ALS. This simply means using any type of light other than sunlight. Needless to say these light examinations must be done at night or beneath a hood or box that blocks out the ambient light.

Each step in this process will be photographed, as will each piece of evidence found. Also, one officer will be assigned to make a written chronology, complete with sketches, of the process. Each item found will be located within the grid on these sketches by measuring its distance from two sides of the grid. This is to record the exact position of each evidence item and its relationship to the area and to other pieces of evidence. Each corpse and any other materials found will be bagged and tagged so that the chain of custody for the evidence will remain intact.

All of these materials will then be transported to the crime lab for analysis.

Can Stored Blood Be Used to Stage a Murder?

Q: If my character banked her blood in preparation for an operation, but the blood was never needed, and then a year later sprinkled it about to make it look like she had been murdered, could anyone tell by analyzing the blood that it wasn't from, as it were, a fresh corpse?

Hallie Ephron
Coauthor of the Dr. Peter Zak mysteries by G. H. Ephron
www.hallieephron.com

A: There are two basic ways the blood could be stored. In both, the blood would have to be refrigerated to prevent decay.

The first way would be to let the blood clot and then store it. Here the age of the blood can be determined to some extent by examining the organization of the clotted blood. What this means is that blood clots by producing protein strands that increase in number as the process continues. These strands give the clot strength, which makes it an effective barrier to further bleeding when you cut your finger. Blood takes about five to fifteen minutes to clot. Over the next several hours, the clot "organizes." This means that these strands contract, pulling it into a tighter bundle, and the fibers appear organized rather than like a bunch of random strands. This strengthens the clot. Under the microscope the age of the clot can be determined to some extent. Not very accurately, but the difference between twelve hours and twelve months would not be difficult to determine. But for your scenario, clotted blood is difficult to "spread around the scene." It would be like using a butter knife to spread Jell-O. Not easy.

The second method would be to store the blood as a liquid. The problem here is that the blood would have to contain an anticoagulant to prevent clotting. Usually this is something like EDTA or heparin. This anticoagulant-containing blood would remain liquid and could be spread around the scene easily. But the problem here is that the blood would remain unclotted forever. That's not what one would expect at a crime scene, where the shed blood should clot in five to fifteen minutes. Once blood has been prevented from coagulating it will not clot on command. The fact that it didn't would cause the ME to test the blood, and the anticoagulant would be found.

Also, the pattern of the blood at the scene is a problem in staging. Forensic experts use the blood-spatter pattern to determine how the blood was spilled, where the victim was at the time, perhaps where the assailant was at the a time, and what weapon or type of blow caused the particular pattern found at the scene. It is a complex process, but it is often crucial to solving a crime and proving or disproving a suspect's or witness's version of the events. Simply pouring or slinging blood around the area would look exactly like it was poured or slung.

So you can see that using stored blood to stage a scene is fraught with problems. That's the bad news. The good news is that all of this is in an ideal world. If your story takes place is a rural location or in a city with an unsophisticated police department, crime lab, and coroner, they may not know the difference between clotted blood and unclotted blood, and may have no experience in crime-scene analysis and re-creation. In which case they would see a bunch of blood and assume someone must have died and press on with that assumption. Happens all the time.

This would be even truer if the blood had soaked a mattress, car seat, carpet, or some other material. In this situation it would be more difficult to characterize the blood as clotted or not. Here they could collect samples, send them away to a lab that would confirm that the blood belonged to the supposed victim (if they had blood or hair or some other DNA source from the supposed victim to compare it with), and determine that the person must indeed be dead due to the sheer volume of blood. This soaking of the blood into a mattress or carpet might even fool a more sophisticated ME and crime lab if they didn't test the blood for anticoagulants, which they might very well not. Why would they suspect a staged scene in the first place? The answer is that they might not.

What volume would be needed? A pint isn't enough, but if the person collected four or five pints of blood (she could give and store a pint a month for four months) and used it all, the police would determine that the mattress held so much blood that the person who shed it could not possibly have survived. They would take a similar mattress and soak it with blood until they achieved a pattern similar to that found at the scene. They could then say how much blood had been shed at the scene, determine that this amount of blood loss was not compatible with survival, declare the person dead, and life would go on.

Was DNA Testing Available in the Early 1990s?

Q: In my mystery a crime must occur just before DNA testing was widely accepted in the United States. How late could that be? Early 1990s, or later?

Lisa King
San Clemente, California
Author of the Jean Applequist mystery series

A: Sir Alec Jeffreys hammered out the DNA profiling technique in 1984 and published his work in *Nature* in 1985. It was first used in a case in England in 1986, the famous Colin Pitchfork case, which was written about by Joseph Wambaugh in his book *The Blooding*. It was first brought to a U.S. civil courtroom in 1986 in *People v. Pestinikas* and to a U.S. criminal courtroom in 1987, where it was used to convict rapist Tommy Lee Andrews in Orlando, Florida. DNA evidence was challenged in 1987 in *New York v. Castro*. This led to a call for some standardization of the DNA procedure, and then to the publication of *DNA Technology in Forensic Science* by the National Research Council Committee on Forensic DNA (NRC I) in 1992 and *The Evaluation of Forensic DNA Evidence* by the second National Research Council Committee on Forensic DNA (NRC II) in 1996. An FBI DNA database (NIDIS) was started in 1998.

In summary, DNA was used as early as 1984, reached the criminal justice system in the United States by 1987, became accepted in 1993, and became widely used sometime between 1993 and 1996.

So the answer to your question is yes. If you set your story in 1993 or earlier, it would work for your needs.

Can Blood and DNA Be Found on a Knife Years Later?

Q: A woman with A negative blood uses a stiletto-type knife to commit suicide. The ambulance crew wipes her blood from the knife, and no special care is taken to preserve the knife and any blood on it. Years later the same knife is used to commit several murders. If the knife is analyzed in a lab, is it possible that the woman's A negative blood from the suicide could still be on the knife and be detectable?

A: Yes, no, maybe. Anything is possible. Often blood is found in the crevices where the blade joins the handle, even if the blade has been thoroughly wiped clean. The perpetrator can't see it and thinks the knife is clean, but in the lab the area is swabbed with a moist Q-tip, and a tiny amount of blood can sometimes be found. Or not. Maybe there is nothing, and the knife really is clean. This means you can write your story either way—yes, there is blood or no, there is not. Either way works.

After the blood is swabbed away, it can be subjected to the DNA techniques of PCR and STR. PCR is polymerase chain reaction, a method to amplify (increase the amount of) any DNA found. This technique simply uses the DNA to reproduce itself until there is enough to use for creating a DNA fingerprint. STR is the technique of using short tandem repeats, a highly sensitive and accurate method for producing the DNA fingerprint.

On the other hand, the DNA could be so degraded that it is unusable; i.e., even though blood was found it is of little help forensically. Acids, heat, and time can damage the DNA and render it unusable.

Also, when the lab analyzes the knife, blood from each of the murders may be found. This will take a bit of work for your forensic serologist (blood expert) to separate out the various blood and DNA types, but it can often be done. This way it might be possible to connect the knife to multiple murders. Or the blood samples may be so numerous and confusing that it is not possible to separate out profiles for each person whose blood is on the knife. Maybe some and not others. Anything is possible.

So you may or may not find blood, and if so it may or may not be useful. This gives you great leeway in crafting your story.

Can Mitochondrial DNA Be Used to Trace the Ancestry of a Man?

Q: I have a question about mitochondrial DNA. Is it only useful for tracing lineage in females, or can males trace their ancestors back centuries, too?

M. Diane Vogt
Tampa, Florida
www.mdianevogt.com

A: Both males and females can trace their ancestry with mito-chondrial DNA (mtDNA), but only through their maternal line. That is, mother, maternal grandmother, maternal great-grandmother, and so on. It will, however, not follow back up the paternal line. That is, the father will have different mtDNA than either his son or daughter. The father's mtDNA will match that of his mother, his maternal grandmother, and so on, but not that of his son. Or his father or grandfather.

Why? Let's look at where we get our mtDNA. The DNA used for standard DNA testing is nuclear DNA. That is, it resides in the nucleus of the cell. This is our genetic DNA in that it contains our inherited genes. But cells also contain nonnuclear DNA. This DNA is found within the mitochondria, which are small organelles that reside within the cytoplasm (the soup) of the cell. The mito-chondria serve as the cell's energy production center. A small amount of DNA is found within each mitochondria, and each cell contains many of these mitochondria organelles. So where do we get our mitochondria?

At fertilization the egg supplies the cell and half the DNA, while the sperm supplies only half the DNA. The sperm cell itself breaks down and disappears after passing its genetic material into the nucleus of the egg cell. This means that all the cell components of the developing zygote come from the mother. This includes the mitochondria. As the cell divides and multiplies, these mitochon-dria are copied and passed on, generation after generation. So a female will pass both nuclear and mtDNA on to her children, while a male will not. He donates nuclear DNA but no mtDNA to his offspring.

Since mtDNA is very stable and only mutates about every sixty-five hundred years, anyone can trace his or her maternal ancestry back thousands of years. But not their paternal ancestry. At least not yet. A newer technique called Y-chromosomal DNA seems to follow the paternal line as mtDNA does the maternal one. It isn't completely hammered out yet, though.

Will Toxicological Testing Reveal That the Victim Was a Chronic Drug User?

Q: Can the ME use a drug screen to determine that a character is a long-term drug user, or would that only come from a physical examination of the liver and/or other organs?

Paula L. Woods
Los Angeles, California
The Charlotte Justice mystery series
www.woodsontheweb.com

A: You are correct. A toxicological screen simply "screens" for the common drugs, and only shows whether they are present in the sample analyzed. More definitive testing is needed to determine the exact drug and the exact level of it in the sample. So a screen may show that an amphetamine is present, and more definitive testing would show which amphetamine (methamphetamine, pseudoephedrine, etc.) was present, and at what levels it was present at the time of death or at the time the sample was taken in the living. But that is all the toxicological testing does.

To show that someone was a chronic user would require evidence of organ or entry-site changes. Common evidence of site variations are scarred veins and a perforated nasal septum. Damage to the liver, lungs, kidneys, or other organs typical for the drug in question will also suggest chronic excessive use. For example, the finding of an elevated blood alcohol level may show that the person is acutely intoxicated, while the finding of alcoholic liver cirrhosis (even if no alcohol is present in the blood at the time of testing) would indicate chronic use.

Toxicological testing shows a slice in time, while the autopsy would show evidence of physical damage from chronic use.

Can a Murder Weapon Be Identified from the Bullet Found at the Crime Scene?

Q: My character owns a .38, is a bit emotionally unstable, and is known to be a good shot. She is seen leaving the scene of a crime where a man has been shot once in the forehead, so she becomes a suspect. If no casing was found at the scene, could an identification of the gun be made with the bullet alone? Is it possible the bullet could have exited so that it isn't found? In the absence of either a casing or a bullet, would forensic investigators be able to rule her gun out as a weapon, or is her goose cooked anyway unless the real killer is found?

Blaize Clement

Sarasota, Florida

Author of the Dixie Hemingway mystery series

www.blaizeclement.com

A: When a gun is fired marks are left on both the bullet and the shell casing. Grooves and striations are cut into the bullet as it spins down the barrel, and on the shell casing as it is slammed backward into the breechblock of the weapon. These markings are very individual and can be used to match the bullet or the shell casing to a particular gun. Of course, matching the crime-scene bullet to a particular gun requires the possession of the suspect gun. It could then be test fired and the bullet or shell casing matched to the ones found at the scene quite accurately. But if the bullet is severely damaged or misshapen from hitting bones or doors or trees it may not be useful for such matching.

Obviously if no bullet or shell casing is found, the examiner will have nothing to compare, even if he has the suspect weapon in hand. In this case it would be your character's gun. But the ME and the forensic firearms examiner may be able to estimate the caliber of a gun by examining the victim's wound. They are often able to distinguish a .22 from a .38 or a .44. Not always, particularly if the wound is angled or irregular, or if the bullet was a hollow point. Hollow-point ammo tends to make much larger wounds than a normal bullet of the same caliber.

This means you can have it either way. Yes, they can tell the caliber, or no they can't. If the wound suggested that the caliber of the murder weapon was larger than your character's .38, such as a .44, or smaller, such as .22, then her weapon would not be the murder weapon. On the other hand, if the caliber of her gun is such that it could have produced the wound, then she isn't off the hook. Regardless, this is only circumstantial evidence, and not very strong circumstantial evidence at that. To prosecute her they would have to match the casing or the bullet to a particular gun.

Yes, the bullet could remain in the corpse, or it could be found in a wall or a tree or somewhere else if it passed through the victim. Or it may not be found at all. If they have an intact bullet or a shell casing they could easily determine the caliber of the weapon.

So a wound, a shell casing, and/or a bullet can often reveal the caliber of the gun used. But to prove which gun of that caliber fired the killing bullet requires matching the bullet or shell casing to a particular weapon.

How Could a Crime-Scene Bullet Be Altered to Render It Unusable as Evidence?

Q: The scenario in my screenplay in progress is that a guy gets shot and killed with a Glock. The bullet is retrieved from the body at autopsy. It is a bit banged up but still in good enough shape for a ballistics match. So the killer's accomplice, who is a cop, contrives to be alone with the bullet for two minutes and uses a hammer to bash the bullet enough to prevent it from being used for matching. Does this make sense? How much banging would he have to do?

Matt Witten
Author of *The Killing Bee*
Supervising producer of the TV show *House*

A: Yes, this could work if the bullet was severely damaged by the hammer. Of course, it would be very obvious that someone had pounded on the bullet. Hammers aren't very subtle.

However, I might make another suggestion. In bullet comparisons it is the surface of the bullet that is critical. This is where the grooves and striations that allow matching are laid down by the barrel's rifling. Anything that altered or added striations to the surface would prevent a match from being made. A file or coarse steel wool or sandpaper or any abrasive material could do this. This way the alteration may not be quite so evident as it would be if a hammer were taken to the bullet, and thus the dirty cop could be home free. Or if you want him to be suspected of altering the bullet, the examiner could find bits of sand or steel wool adhering to the bullet and suspect that something had been used on it. Also, some of the new microscopic scratches would not be exactly parallel to the long axis of the bullet, as the striations made during travel down the barrel are. Either of these findings would suggest a later alteration.

Is It Possible to Determine if Bruises on a Corpse Occurred Before or After Death?

Q: A man is pushed into San Francisco Bay and his body is recovered forty-eight hours later, beneath a pier. There are some contusions to the head, either from the person who killed him or from knocking against the pier. Will the ME be able to determine if the contusions were made before or after death?

> Lisa King
> San Clemente, California
> Author of the Jean Applequist mystery series

A: Most likely the ME would be able to determine if the bruises occurred before or after death. The simple reason is that it is very difficult to bruise a corpse. Let me explain.

Contusions (bruises) result from damage to the small blood vessels in the tissues. These injured vessels then leak blood, which imparts a blue-black color to the injured area. If the blood collects in a pocket beneath the skin (goose egg) it is called a hematoma. *Heme* means blood and *toma* means tumor. So a hematoma is a tumor, or mass of blood.

Since a bruise takes several minutes to appear, if the victim suffers a contusing blow many minutes or hours before death, the resulting bruise will be fairly diffuse and widespread around the area of impact. However, if the blow is struck perimortem (around the time of death), the bruise will be smaller and more clearly defined. The perimortem period may be defined as seconds or a very few minutes before or after death. Why are perimortem bruises smaller? It takes time for the blood to seep into and spread through the tissues. If death interrupts this process, the bruise will be smaller and have more distinct edges.

What about postmortem contusions? Is it possible to bruise a corpse? Yes, but it's difficult. Since a contusion depends upon a leakage of blood from injured vessels, it should be obvious that a bruise requires that blood be flowing into the injured vessel. At death the heart stops, the blood ceases to circulate, and blood clotting occurs in a few minutes. Any injury to the vessel after death would not produce a bruise. That said, if a blow to a corpse is delivered with sufficient force, vessels may be severely damaged and blood may leak into the area of impact. In this situation the ME may not be able to determine if the blow was premortem or postmortem.

Sometimes a body suspected of having suffered blunt-force trauma shows no evidence of bruising on the surface. This may be the case if the bruising has occurred deeply within the tissues and muscles and if the victim did not live long enough for the bruising to seep to the surface. In this situation, during the autopsy, the ME may make a series of deep cuts into the muscles and down to the bones, along the back, arms, and legs, in a search for deep bruising. He will also look for contusions of internal organs such as the liver, heart, lungs, and brain.

The ME must examine contusions carefully and determine if they occurred pre-, peri-, or postmortem. He must also determine if any of the contusing blows were potentially lethal, since these determinations can directly affect the cause and time of death as well as substantiate or refute a suspect's account of events.

Was Semen Useful for Determining Blood Type in 1939?

Q: In 1939, could homicide detectives in a Midwestern American state determine a suspect's blood type from semen deposited on the body of a murder victim?

Susan Vercellino
Associate Producer
James B. Harris Productions

A: Most likely yes.

Karl Landsteiner (1868–1943) discovered the four basic blood types in 1901, and in 1930 was awarded the Nobel Prize for his work. In 1925 it was found that 80 percent of individuals were "secretors." This means that they secrete proteins identical to those in their blood into other bodily fluids, such as semen, saliva, and tears. Thus a man with blood type A would secrete type A antigens (proteins) into his semen. Nonsecretors have their blood-type antigens in their blood but not in these other fluids. So by 1939 the existence of secretors and nonsecretors was known.

Also, as a consequence of the famous St. Valentine's Day Massacre on February 14, 1929, the first private crime lab was established at Northwestern University in Chicago.

This means that by 1939 the necessary science had been established and the Midwest had a multiservice crime lab. This knowledge could easily have reached the locale of your story, and your crack coroner could submit the samples to Northwestern's lab, the FBI (which soon thereafter developed its own labs), or a regional fictional lab of your creation. Any of these labs could use the semen sample to determine the perpetrator's blood type.

How Would the Condition of the Corpse of Someone Who Froze to Death in a Freezer Differ from That of Someone Who Froze on a Remote Mountain?

Q: How would the effects on a body be different in a person who died in a commercial or home freezer from one who died from exposure to the elements on a mountain where the low temperature was 28 degrees? Would the effects of alcohol in the man's system alter the circumstances?

Dale E. Sperling
Author of *The Queen of Southgate*

A: In either situation the body could be completely frozen, and thus would be very well preserved. There would be two major areas of difference between the exposed and the protected corpse.

The temperature in a commercial freezer and most high-quality home freezers is well below 28 degrees, particularly in the commercial ones, generally in the range between 10 degrees below zero and 10 degrees Fahrenheit. Also, the temperature in either would remain steady, and the corpse could be well preserved for many years. In nature the temperature varies greatly, and there may be times when the temperature is above freezing. This would allow for some thawing of the body on the surface, if nowhere else. This in turn would allow for some bacterial growth and some degree of decay to take hold. This means that the exposed body would be more decayed than the one in the freezer. In this case the putrefaction process would be over the surface of the corpse, with the central parts being preserved. This is in contrast to the typical decay pattern, which occurs from the inside out.

Other areas of difference are the weather and predators. Rain and sleet could damage the body, particularly if it were washed down a stream or if water flowed over it. Predators will feed on bodies if they can get to them. These predators range from insects to carnivores such as dogs, cats, wolves, and others. They can consume portions of the corpse and scatter parts far and wide. Obviously a frozen corpse would be less appetizing to them than a fresh kill would be, but in winter they take what they can get, and gnawing on a frozen corpse is better than starving.

The bottom line is that the corpse in the freezer will be very well preserved while the one exposed to the elements may or may not be.

The amount of alcohol in the blood in even a severely intoxicated individual is negligible and would alter the course of decay or preservation little if any.

What Would a Body Look Like After Five Years in a Periodically Frozen Swamp?

Q: A body is dumped in a shallow, northern wilderness swamp, which is frozen for roughly six months of the year. Otherwise the climate is very variable. What condition would this body be in after five years?

> Shelley Costa
> Chagrin Falls, Ohio
> 2004 Edgar Award nominee (short story category)

A: Corpses can undergo several different types of alteration over time. Putrefaction (decay), mummification, and adipocere formation are the common ones, with putrefaction being by far the most frequently seen.

Most likely the corpse would be a skeleton. Though frozen for six months each year, the remainder of the year the body would be subject to warmer weather conditions. This would allow for thawing and would expose the corpse to predators and putrefaction. Each spring and summer the body would decay a little more, until there was no tissue left, only bones, teeth, and perhaps hair.

It is possible that if the swamp area is very acidic, which happens during the decay of various plants and plant parts that fall into the water, the corpse or portions of it could be mummified, as is seen with "bog people" (mummies found in bogs). This occurs because the acidic nature of the water kills bacteria and therefore prevents decay. In this circumstance the corpse could be remarkably well preserved. Facial features and fingerprints might be spared, and it might even be possible to extract DNA from the tissues.

The third thing that could happen to the corpse in this circumstance is adipocere formation. Adipocere is a whitish-gray waxy substance that forms when body fat is exposed to certain conditions, such as an acidic environment. Since fat is spread throughout the body, this adipocere formation can occur everywhere, and the corpse would look eerily like a wax doll. Spooky.

And in some situations all three are seen in the same corpse. Some parts might be skeletonized, some mummified, and others could form adipocere. For example, the head could be adipocere, the chest and arms mummified, and the lower extremities skeletal. Or any other combination. It's unpredictable. Still, the most likely result is that the corpse would a skeleton.

Does a Buried Body Have an Odor After Twelve Hours?

Q: My story takes place in the Los Angeles area in April. A body that lay dead in a building for about twelve hours is then buried in a shallow grave and discovered about eight hours after burial. The temperature is 50 to 60 degrees or so. Would the corpse's odor be strong enough that my character might detect it while walking nearby?

Sybil A. Johnson
Manhattan Beach, California

A: Actually, under the conditions you describe, there would be very little odor, only a faint musty or rotten one, and it would likely go unnoticed until the body was uncovered. The odor of a corpse comes from putrefaction (decay), which is caused by bacteria. Much like leaving meat out on a countertop. Actually, exactly like that. Bacteria like moist, warm environments. After twelve hours a body in a garage in Houston in August would be well into the decay process and would smell, but with an ambient temperature of only 50 to 60 degrees, it would not. Under these conditions it could be as much as 48 to 96 hours before the odor attracted the attention of anyone passing by. This is particularly true with a buried corpse, even if the grave is shallow.

This means that your character would likely have to have some other means of stumbling on the body, since odor would be an unlikely clue. Perhaps a dog had dug into the ground and exposed a hand or foot, or maybe an article of clothing was left nearby. When your character investigated he would find that the ground had been disturbed and might then notice the faint odor of decay.

What Would a Corpse That Had Been Buried Beneath Concrete for Five Months Look Like?

Q: If a body were buried under cement, would bloodhounds pick up the scent? How would that body look after five months in the ground? Would the coroner be able to determine the cause of death? Injuries to the skull? Bruising around the neck? I assume the police would wait for an ME to touch/remove the body? Any special care needed to move the body? Any techniques?

> Rochelle Krich
> Mary Higgins Clark Award–winning author of *Grave Endings* and *Now You See Me . . .*
> www.rochellekrich.com

A: There are several possibilities here. What the corpse looked like would depend for the most part on how well the body is preserved, and this in turn would depend upon how deeply the body was buried, how much concrete overlay it, what the nature of the soil was, and what the ambient temperature and level of moisture was.

Warm, moist soil would favor bacterial growth, and thus putrefaction. If putrefaction progressed rapidly, only skeletal remains would be found. Cadaver dogs would be less likely to pick up a scent, since they key on the odor of decaying flesh. The ME could determine bone and skull damage but not tissue injury in this circumstance. He still might be able to state that strangulation was the cause of death if the hyoid bone (a small bone in the neck) had been fractured during the assault. Of course, he would have to take into consideration the weight of the cement, which may have fractured this delicate bone too.

On the other hand, if the conditions were very cool and dry, the body might be fairly well preserved. Here the cadaver dogs would be more likely to pick up a scent, and the ME would have both bones and tissues to work with. He might find the above-mentioned bony injuries as well as signs of bruising, stabbing, cutting, and whatever other trauma the victim might have suffered.

And there could be anything in between these two extremes. The body could be partially skeletonized and partially preserved. The dogs could or could not pick up the scent. The ME could or could not see bruises. The fractures of the skull and the hyoid bone could or could not lead him to say that the victim was struck and/or strangled.

So for your scenario this uncertainty would work well. You can have the findings fit any of these and they would be possible and believable.

Yes, the ME or one of his assistants would come to the site. The body would be photographed in situ (as it is), trace evidence would be searched for, and the body would be placed on and wrapped in plastic for transportation, which is routine. Then the underlying and surrounding soil would be examined, and maybe even collected into bags so it could later be sifted for trace evidence at the lab.

Can Eye Movements Reveal That Someone Is Lying?

Q: Is it true that when someone lies during an interrogation he will subconsciously move his eyes to the left and when recalling something from memory he will look to the right? If this is true, can my character tell lies while suppressing this subconscious behavior?

Dion Debono

Malta

A: First of all, there are no foolproof signs of deception. Humans are simply too diverse in their reactions to stress. Some people are shy or nervous by nature and will show signs of stress under almost any circumstance. Some sociopaths can lie at will and show absolutely no stress. And anything in between. This is why lie detectors (polygraphs) are rarely admitted in court.

What you are describing is called neurolinguistic programming (NLP). It is a theory that certain eye movements reflect certain mental processes.

Briefly, the theory of NLP is that deflection of the eyes mirror what the person is undergoing mentally. Eyes directed up and to the right mean the person is recalling something he has seen, while up and to the left means he is constructing a new mental image. To the right side (toward his right ear) or downward and to the right, he is remembering something he has heard, while to the left side (toward his left ear) he is creating a new auditory mental construct. Down and to the left he is recalling certain feelings or smells.

Based on this, if someone is asked a question and looks up and to the right while answering, he is describing something that he has seen before. Perhaps the crime scene? Or maybe the victim? If he looks up and to the left, he is creating an image on the fly and could be lying, or perhaps is creating the image he thinks his questioner wants him to. Regardless, in the latter instance he never really saw what he says he saw.

The same is true with looking to the right or left for things he heard or says he heard.

That's the theory anyway. Neither NLP nor any of the other physical clues are absolute or universal. Like stop signs in Italy, they are merely suggestions.

If your character knew about NLP and thought his interrogator might also know and use the technique, he could simply force himself to look the opposite way, or at his own lap, or stare the questioner directly in the eyes. The eye movements described above are subconscious and can be overridden with conscious effort. At least for a while. As the interrogation stretched on he might fatigue and fall into subconscious responses.

What Methods Exist for Exposing Second-Page Writing?

Q: In my story I need for my detective to uncover the contents of a note from the indentions left on the next page of the pad it was written on. What are the different ways these impressions can be exposed?

A: This second-page writing is called "indented writing," since the movement of the pen over the top page indents the second along the path of the pen. I'm sure you've taken a pencil and, using the side of the lead, rubbed it back and forth over the surface of the second page and seen the "invisible" writing appear. Though this works, forensic technicians don't use this method, since the pencil's markings might destroy or damage the evidence. It would at least alter it and likely make it inadmissible in court. So techniques that do not damage or alter the page are used.

Sometimes a simple angled light will reveal indented writing. Here the indentions, when exposed to an acutely angled light, will produce shadows that reveal the indented writing. This is exactly like the shadows that appear and deepen in low-lying areas as the sun descends toward the horizon. The page can then be photographed.

A more sensitive method is the use of an electrostatic detection apparatus (ESDA). This is a highly sensitive technique that can expose even the faintest of indentions, and can on occasion uncover indented writing several pages below the original page. It's interesting that no one knows exactly how ESDA works, only that it does.

With ESDA the page in question is covered with a Mylar sheet and placed on a porous metal plate. A vacuum is applied, which pulls the Mylar tightly against the page. The Mylar is to protect the page, which is potential evidence, against damage. Static electricity is produced in the Mylar sheet-page combination by passing an electric wand over them. Though this process charges the entire surface of the Mylar, the charge is greatest in any indentions on the page. Black toner similar to that used in copy machines is poured or sprayed over the Mylar. It attaches to the surface in proportion to the degree of charge, which means that the indentions retain the greatest concentration of the toner. This reveals the indentions, and thus the writing.

Can the Language Used in an E-Mail Be Used to Determine Authorship?

Q: Is there a recognized linguistic technique to analyze patterns of written language, and therefore determine authorship? For example, could e-mails sent anonymously be compared with other written material of known authorship, and a connection established/suggested? I am working on a story where a pivotal character exerts influence solely through e-mail/Internet chat rooms. Could my suspect be identified by such techniques?

> Craig Vicary
> Leuven, Belgium

A: Absolutely. Forensic document examiners do exactly this. They not only look at the writing itself and analyze hard-copy paper and ink chemically, but also attempt to profile the writer as to education, ethnic background, writing style, type of employment, and other things. This linguistic analysis is done whether the document is handwritten, typed, photocopied, or on a computer printout, and whether it is a letter, ransom or bank robbery note, altered contract, or writing on a bathroom wall.

And this is not new. It was used in famous cases such as the

Mormon Murders and the Hitler diaries forgery cases, as well as for the Lindbergh kidnapping case, known as the crime of the century. When the son of Colonel Charles Lindbergh was abducted from the family home in Hopewell, New Jersey, on the night of March 1, 1932, five years after the "Lone Eagle" became the first person to fly solo across the Atlantic, the kidnapper left a ransom note. Examination of the note revealed no fingerprints, but the language used led investigators to conclude that the abductor was poorly educated and likely of German descent. Bruno Hauptmann, who was ultimately convicted and executed for the crime, matched this profile.

To help identify the author of various types of documents, the FBI maintains several databases. These include the National Fraudulent Check File, the Bank Robbery Note File, and the Anonymous Letter File.

With e-mails, the document examiner would work with forensic computer experts and attempt to track their origin, and would also analyze the wording for all of the above. Of course, handwriting and ink and paper analysis would play no role here, which makes the analysis of the words and sentences and phrases used all that more important. When successful, the determination of ethnicity, education, writing style, and a guess as to the writer's age, sex, region of residence, employment, religion, and political beliefs can narrow the search for the perpetrator greatly.

Is It Possible for My Sleuth to Determine That Hair and Fiber Evidence from a Crime Scene Was Planted?

Q: I'm toying with having my criminal plant hair and fiber evidence on a victim to implicate my crime solver. Since my stories are set in a high-tech manufacturing environment, all parties involved are well trained in how to control particulate contamination. The murder doesn't actually take place there, however. How would my crime solver figure out that the evidence was planted? I can have him trick the criminal into revealing it, but I wondered if the evidence itself would in any way indicate that it was planted.

Arlene Sachitano

Portland, Oregon

Author of *Chip and Die,* a Harley Spring mystery

A: This is a tough one. Your sleuth may or may not be able to do this. The key would be to find the fibers in a location where they would not be expected to be, based on the reconstruction of the crime scene. A classic example is the famous Jeffrey MacDonald case. He was a Green Beret physician in North Carolina who murdered his wife and two children, claiming that a group of "hippies" had broken in and knocked him unconscious in the living room after he struggled with them, and that they tore his blue cotton pajama top. They then proceeded to the bedrooms and killed his family while he was out. However, crime-scene analysis turned up numerous fibers from his pajamas in the bedroom where his wife was killed, some fibers where the children were killed, and almost none in the living room. This meant that the top was likely torn in his bedroom, and was probably done in a struggle with his wife. Thus, the location and number of the fibers contradicted his account.

In your scenario, when your perpetrator stages the crime scene, he would place the fibers on or near the victim, so they would be found, and the wrong person would become a suspect. Your sleuth could find some of the fibers and hairs clumped or twisted together in an odd way, and might say that the natural falling away of hair and fiber would not produce this. He might suspect that someone had sprinkled them around the victim.

Or your perpetrator could accidentally drop some of the hair and fibers at the wrong place. For example, he might break a window so the police would think that this was the point of entry, and then leave a rear door ajar so that this would look like the point of exit. But some of the fibers could be found near another door— the true point of entry and exit—and this could raise an eyebrow or two. Criminals usually have only one point of entry and one point of exit. Having a third area come into play would be odd.

This oddity might make your sleuth dig a little deeper and give him a rational motive for tricking the perpetrator into telling the truth.

For a Victim of a Gunshot to the Head, Is It Possible for the Coroner to Determine if the Body Was Moved an Hour After Death?

Q: The victim of a gunshot to the head is found on a back porch. If the body is moved an hour after death would the ME be able to detect that fact? The weapon is a .22 caliber pistol, and there is a small entrance wound in one temple, but no exit wound. Could a .22 bullet lodge in the skull?

> Carolyn Hart
> Oklahoma City, Oklahoma
> Author of *Dead Days of Summer*

A: First let's look at the bullet. It's not only possible but likely that a small caliber bullet such as a .22 would not pass completely through the skull, and would remain lodged somewhere in the brain. It could exit or it could not, so you can write your scene however you want.

Could the ME determine if the body had been moved? Maybe, maybe not. Lividity is often used to determine if a body has been repositioned or relocated. Lividity (also called livor mortis) is the dark blue-gray discoloration of the dependent (lower) areas of a corpse, and is due to a settling of the blood in the vessels. If the body is lying on its back, the settling will be along the back, the back of the head, and the back of the legs. If the body is rolled to one side, the settling will occur along that side. For the first four hours or so the lividity can be shifted in this manner, and as you might guess this is called "shifting" lividity. This means that a body lying on its back will begin to show lividity along the back. If it is rolled to the right side a couple of hours later, the lividity will shift and begin to collect on that side. But after four to eight hours this blood seeps out of the vessels and stains the tissues. The result is that the lividity is now fixed, so that moving the corpse to a different position will not shift the discoloration. This is called "fixed" lividity. So if the ME saw that the corpse had lividity along the back, yet the victim was lying facedown, he would conclude that the corpse had been moved. And since a corpse can't move on its own, someone was there to move it.

But in your scenario, where the body is moved after only an hour, this is of no use, since this is not enough time for any lividity to appear, much less become fixed. Unless you forward this timeline, that is. If you have the body lie in one position for about six hours before it is moved, you can use the lividity pattern to help your investigators.

But the bleeding pattern might be useful in this regard. For example, if the victim were shot at the location and in the position he was found, the ME would expect to find the high-velocity blood-spatter pattern that is typical of gunshots on the floor, the wall, nearby furniture, and any other object in the immediate area. If he did not see this he might suspect that the person had been shot somewhere else. Of course, the small-caliber .22 may not produce much spatter anyway, and he might simply write it off to that.

Or let's say the victim is found lying on his left side, and this is the same side as the entry wound. Let's further say that blood from the wound had oozed across his face and down his chin. Since blood will not ooze or flow uphill (against gravity) this finding would mean that the victim had been lying on his right side after being shot, and was then rolled over to his other side. Otherwise the blood would have simply leaked onto the floor and not across his face.

I should point out that the amount of blood would depend upon how quickly the victim died. Since dead folks don't bleed, blood loss would cease when his heart stopped. This could be almost instantly, or it could be several hours later. All gunshots to the brain are not immediately fatal, contrary to what is portrayed in the movies. In fact, many people live to reach the ER, and even survive. If he died quickly there would be little bleeding, but if he lived for a period of time there would be more.

Will a Corpse Left in a House for Many Months Mummify?

Q: I want to have a character in my novel die of natural causes. She will waste away from cancer, and die emaciated and dehydrated at home in bed. And then just remain there, unburied. (Think Norman Bates's mother in *Psycho*.) Is this at all conceivable? Would the neighbors notice a smell or a swarm of flies? Could anything be done to the body so it would dry up and become mummified? How long would it smell, and what would it be like a year later?

Hallie Ephron
Coauthor of the Dr. Peter Zak mysteries by G. H. Ephron
www.hallieephron.com

A: Yes, this can happen, and indeed it does from time to time. Often isolated people will die at home and not be found for weeks, months, even years. These corpses can be partially decayed, skeletonized, or mummified, depending upon conditions and luck. "Whatever happens, happens" is the rule here.

Decay or putrefaction is favored in warm, humid environments (bacteria thrive under these conditions). If the putrefaction continues, the tissues of the corpse will be completely consumed, and only a skeleton will remain. Colder and drier climes favor mummification. Also, hot and dry climes can desiccate (dry out) a corpse, which will lead to mummy formation. And a given corpse can be a combination of these processes. That is, a corpse may be partially mummified and partially skeletonized.

The odor of decay results from the gases produced by the bacteria, and the odor would linger for as long as it takes for the tissues to decay completely. In an enclosed structure the odor may be well contained, and neighbors or the mailman or anyone knocking on the door might not notice anything. Depending upon conditions, the corpse could decay completely in a week or two, or over several months. In a swamp in Florida, a week or so could be long enough, while in a house in the Midwest it could take many weeks or months. Also in an enclosed room, flies would not be a major problem, as they are around corpses in exposed areas, though they could appear. Again, if no one entered the house they wouldn't know whether a swarm of flies was in one of the rooms or not.

For your scenario a hot and dry region such as Arizona would be best for mummification, but this could still happen in Norman's mother's house, or any other house for that matter. The fact that your victim was severely dehydrated before death would make mummification even more likely.

This means that you can have your corpse mummify and no one would know until someone went inside to check things out. Or the corpse could decay completely, leaving behind skeletal remains, and again no one would know until they entered the home.

If you wanted someone to help the mummification process along, they could pour salt over the corpse. The ancient Egyptians used oils and salts to help dry out the corpse and to prevent decay, and thus produce a mummy, which was their goal. Salt not only helps desiccate the body, it is also a powerful antibacterial agent. Bacteria need moisture to grow, and a high concentration of salt is lethal to bacteria. Salt curing of meat has been used as a method of preservation for centuries, and that's basically what this would be.

Once a body was mummified or skeletonized it would remain basically unchanged for many years, so after a year it would look very much as it did after a month or two—after the putrefaction or mummification process was complete. A mummified corpse is usually dark in color, with the skin pulled tightly over the bones, as if it had been shrink-wrapped. The face would appear to be grimacing, and the eyes would be dried into small dark knots that would be difficult to see, so that the eye sockets would appear to be empty. Creepy. Like Norman.

Can the Type of Sand Found on a Corpse Be Used to Determine the Location of the Murder?

Q: Can a lab differentiate beach sand from one location from that of another? In my story a corpse is found on a California beach. It appears to have been moved. If the sand on the corpse is different from the sand on the beach where it is found, can the sand be matched to the area thirty miles away where the murder actually took place?

Katie McLaughlin
Santa Maria, California

A: It might be possible. It depends upon how much the sand and the environment of the specific areas along the beach vary from one location to another.

The sand along beaches can vary in grain size, shape, color, and refractive and reflective properties (how light bends or bounces off the grains). Sand is a silicate, and there are many types of silicates, which means that sands from different areas may vary in their chemical makeups. Sometimes these physical and chemical properties can be used to determine if a specific sample came from a specific site. Sometimes not.

Also tiny, even microscopic, plant and animal life will vary from location to location, and a forensic botanist can often determine where a specific sample came from. One area may have trees nearby while another has wildflowers. The leaves, needles, seeds, and pollens from these would be mixed with the nearby sand. Certain birds may nest in one area and not in another, and their feathers, nesting materials, or droppings may be found in the sand of one place but not at another ten miles up the road.

If your examiner found pine pollen, pine needles, and tiny plant materials or bird feathers—attached to the corpse or mixed with the sand on the corpse—that weren't native to that area, and if he found that the sand was physically and chemically different from the sand that surrounded the corpse, he could say that the body likely was moved. If he could then match these findings to sand thirty miles up the coast he could at least say that that area was compatible with the scene of the murder, or at least that the body had been there at some prior time.

Another tool you might be able to use is plant DNA. Just like humans, plants have cells, and their cells have DNA. If plant materials were found on the corpse, and if an area up the coast was suspected of being the murder site, plant DNA might help. Let's say your sleuth finds an area beneath a tree where shoeprints or tire tracks or anything suggested that the murder had taken place beneath that tree. And let's also say that the ME found bits of leaves, a few seeds, or some pollen on the corpse. A DNA match between the tree and the materials on the victim would prove that the body and the tree had been close to one another at some time. That connection might solve the crime.

How Is Heroin Detected in the Body?

Q: For my story I need to know how to test a substance to see if it indeed is heroin and what the procedure would involve. What type of lab equipment is used; how long does it take to get the results; and how much of the substance should be tested at a time?

A: The test procedure depends upon whether the lab is given a sample of the chemical, or fluids and tissues from a person or a corpse.

Heroin (diacetylmorphine) is an opiate. Opiates are chemicals that are derived from the sap of the poppy. They are divided into natural, semisynthetic, and synthetic, depending upon their source and method of manufacture. They are narcotic sedatives (sleep producing) and analgesics (pain relieving) that produce euphoria, lethargy, and, in larger doses, coma and death from respiratory depression and asphyxia. Most can be taken either by mouth or injection, and all have great potential for abuse.

Natural opiates come directly from the poppy. Morphine and codeine are the basic ones, and heroin is derived easily from morphine. Semisynthetic opiates are created by making molecular alterations to morphine and codeine. Many medical analgesics are of this type. Hydrocodone, oxymorphone, and oxycodone (OxyContin) are examples. Synthetic opiates are constructed in a laboratory and are not derived from either morphine or codeine. Examples include meperidine (Demerol) and fentanyl.

When heroin is injected, it is almost immediately converted into monoacetylmorphine, which is further converted into morphine. This happens in a matter of minutes. So when someone—living or dead—is tested for heroin, they are actually tested for monoacetylmorphine and morphine, since no heroin will be detected. These substances can be found in the blood, urine, and bile. Testing is easy and can be done in a few hours.

Testing a drug sample for opiates utilizes one of the many chromatographic techniques, such as gas chromatography (GC). These separate the chemicals present, and then with mass spectrometry (MS) each component chemical can be identified. MS identifies a chemical "fingerprint" of any compound, and is very specific.

If blood or other bodily fluids are analyzed, the first step is a screening test for opiates. A commonly used one is the Marquis test, in which the sample is exposed to the Marquis reagent, which is a combination of formaldehyde and sulfuric acid. It turns purple in the presence of opiates. Also, either GC or thin layer chromatography (TLC) can be used in the screening process. If opiates are found, the blood is then subjected to MS and the particular opiate, in your scenario heroin, is identified.

Can Mercury Be Found in a Murder Victim's Hair a Year After Death?

Q: In my mercury poisoning story the victim dies and is buried. A year later my sleuth suspects something is not right with the victim's demise. In fact, she suspects that arsenic might be involved. Is there any way of deter-

mining that he died of mercury poisoning without
exhuming his corpse?

Gay Toltl Kinman
Alhambra, California
Author of *Castle Reiner* and *Super Sleuth: Five Alison
Leigh Powers Mysteries*
gaykinman.com

A: Mercury and arsenic are both heavy metals, as are lead, bismuth, antimony, and thallium. These metals tend to accumulate
within the tissues, and in the hair of the victim if the exposure is
chronic. If the victim died from a single large dose, then exhuming
the body would be necessary. The mercury would then be found in
any remaining tissues. But if the exposure were more chronic, over
weeks or months, then the mercury would also accumulate in the
victim's hair. Here an exhumation may not be needed.

Hair will contain mercury only if the blood level of mercury is
high at the time the hair is formed. In an acute poisoning the victim may die in hours or days, and there just isn't time for hair to
grow. But if the exposure is more chronic, then the hair of the victim will have time to grow, and any growth that takes place in the
presence of mercury will contain mercury.

The only way to discover that the victim was indeed exposed to
mercury without exhuming the body would be to have a sample
of the victim's hair that was taken before death. Maybe a lock was
removed before the funeral and placed in a keepsake book. This
way the killer, if a family member, would unknowingly save the
evidence that could convict him. Irony at its best. Also, hair could
be taken from the hairbrush the victim used before death, or perhaps from some of his saved clothing. The hair could then be
tested, and if found to have a very high level of mercury, the
specter of murder by poisoning would be raised.

The screening tests used for identifying heavy metals include the
Reinsch test or one of several colorimetric tests. These will be positive if any of the heavy metals are present. The toxicologist would
then use either atomic absorption spectrophotometry or neutron
activation analysis to identify which one was present and in what

amount. If the levels were high, an exhumation would be done and the body itself tested.

Can the Instrument Used to Cut a Blanket Be Identified?

Q: Can the instrument used to cut a flannel blanket be identified by careful inspection? This is critical to my plot.

Michelle Graham

A: Probably not the specific instrument but maybe the type of instrument used. This is the domain of the forensic tool mark examiner. He would look at the cut edges of the fibers under a microscope, and perhaps a scanning electron microscope (SEM), and might be able to determine some of the characteristics of the cutting instrument: the sharpness of the blade; the angle of the blade's bevel; whether there was one (knife) or two (scissors) cutting edges; whether the edge was straight or not (pinking shears); whether the blade was smooth or saw-toothed (the latter would fray the edges while the former would make a clean cut); and a few other things. Based on these findings he might be able to state that the instrument was of a certain type. That is, he might be able to say that the cuts were made with scissors as opposed to a knife.

If he had the suspect instrument he could then cut some identical material, and if the cuts matched microscopically, he could state that the instrument could not be excluded as the instrument used to cut the material. And if the blade had a chip missing or some defect and he could match that to a defect in the cut, he could be even more convinced that the instrument in question was the one that made the cut. That's about as far as he could go. He could not say that this exact instrument was the one that made the cut. This type of examination is not specific enough for that.

But if the blade or blades were stained with some chemical or paint or, better yet, blood, and if some of this were deposited on the blanket, then these would add even more individuality, and his confidence would be higher still. And in the case of blood he might be able to make a DNA match, and then he could say that this was the device used. At least the suspect would have to explain how the victim's blood got on his knife or scissors.

How Can Certificates of Birth and Death and DNA Be Used to Prove Parenthood?

Q: How would my sleuth determine that a birth certificate had been falsified? The scenario is that the names recorded are not the birth parents' but rather those of the "adoptive" parents. If the biological parents are told their infant is dead, would a death certificate, or rather the lack of one, prove the child is alive? Who can get copies of birth and death certificates? If a child has been dead and buried for a year or more, what tests can be done to verify the infant's parentage?

Kelly-Lynne Reimer
Winnipeg, Manitoba, Canada

A: Birth and death certificates are records, and as such are subject to all the problems associated with any other documents. They can be destroyed, stolen, altered, or forged. This means that for plot purposes you can use any of these as background for your false documentation. So yes, the adoptive parents' names could appear on the "official" certificate.

The absence of or the inability to locate a specific certificate is not uncommon, and doesn't mean the victim is still alive. Though the appropriate certificate should accompany every birth and every death, this is not always the case. Bureaucracies notoriously screw up these types of things. These records are typically maintained by the county at the courthouse, or wherever the county keeps its records. A birth certificate can be obtained by the person himself, by his parents (unless adoption is involved, and these laws are completely crazy and vary widely from state to state and situation to situation), or by court order. Family, insurance companies, the courts, and many other people can obtain a death certificate. And, of course, an insider can pilfer them or a thief can break in and take them. If they are maintained on computers (this also varies greatly from place to place), the records can be hacked and stolen or altered.

The best test for determining parenthood from remains is DNA. It is extremely accurate, falling in the 99-plus percent range. Of course, DNA must be available in the corpse. If the child had been embalmed and the corpse is mostly intact, DNA should be readily available. If the remains are skeletal, DNA can often be obtained from bone cells and from dental pulp. It only takes a very small amount. The DNA fingerprint of the remains is then determined and compared with those of the parents, and if they match, parenthood is confirmed.

Now a little about DNA:

Through the union of egg and sperm, each parent donates half of his or her DNA to the new child. Neither donates all his or her DNA, however. Remember that our forty-six chromosomes are arranged in twenty-three pairs, and each parent only donates one chromosome of each pair to the child. That way the child also has forty-six chromosomes, twenty-three from each parent. Thus, the child is a combination of the DNA donated by each parent. The parents may have DNA that the child doesn't have (DNA on the chromosome not donated via the egg or sperm), but the child absolutely can't possess DNA that one of the parents didn't donate. This means that when the child's DNA is fragmented and separated into bands (fingerprinted—looks like a bar code), each of the resulting bands must also be found in one or the other parent.

In your scenario, if the remains possess a DNA fragment that is not present in either the suspected mother or father, then one or both of them is not the child's parent. This fragment must have come from someone else (the real father or mother), and parenthood is excluded. If all the bands in the remains match bands in one or the other parent, they are the parents.

Was It Possible to Match a Bullet to a Particular Weapon in the 1980s?

Q: In the 1980s was the field of ballistics advanced enough to match a bullet from a deer rifle to the rifle after the bullet had passed through an unfortunate victim and embedded in a tree trunk? And could hairs from a pointer (dog) be matched with those clinging to someone's clothing?

Charles Schaeffer
Author of stories for *The Storyteller, The Crimson Dagger,* and other publications

A: Such examinations are called firearms examinations, and they have been done since the 1920s. In fact, the case that brought this process to the forefront of forensics was Al Capone's famous St. Valentine's Day Massacre.

On February 14, 1929, Al Capone sent three gunmen dressed as Chicago police officers to visit a bootlegging warehouse run by his rival, George "Bugs" Moran. The men used Thompson submachine guns (Tommy guns) to massacre seven of Bugs's men. Evidence at the scene and from the autopsies gave the police seventy shell casings and as many bullets to work with. Cardiologist and firearms expert Calvin Goddard was brought in to examine the evidence, and he matched the bullets and shell casings to two Tommy guns found at the home of one of Capone's hit men. The handling of this massive amount of evidence and the solving of this famous crime inspired two businessmen who had sat on the coroner's jury to establish the first independent crime lab in the United States. This lab served as the prototype for many future labs. So firearms examination was an established forensic technique long before the 1980s.

Rifling is the grooves cut into the inside of the barrel of rifles and handguns. These grooves impart spin to the bullet, which greatly increases accuracy. When a bullet travels down a rifled barrel, striations are etched into the sidewall of the bullet. The matching of a crime-scene bullet to a specific weapon depends upon the visual comparison of the striations on the crime-scene bullet with those on a test-fired one. It should be obvious that such comparisons require that the crime-scene bullet be in good condition. If it is mangled or severely misshapen, the striations may not be readily visible and a comparison may not be possible. If the bullet is well preserved, a match is usually easy. In your scenario the bullet may be intact or may be severely damaged by its encounters with bones and/or trees, which means you can construct your scene either way and it will work.

Animal hairs can be matched through microscopic visual inspection, but this is much less specific than bullet examination. The examiner may be able to determine the breed, and may be able to say that the hairs match, and that it is likely that they came from the dog in question or from a similar dog. But it cannot be determined that the hair came from a specific dog. This means that, by itself, an animal hair comparison, like human hair and clothing or carpet fibers, is not specific enough to convict, but as part of a circumstantial case, which most are, it can be added evidence against the suspect.

Could the Police or Crime-Scene Investigators Distinguish Murder from an Accidental Death Caused by the Laceration of an Artery by a Quilting Tool?

Q: My victim is killed by a quilting tool, which is a rotary cutter similar to a pizza cutter. It is used to cut through layers of fabric quickly and accurately. My scenario is that the blade nicks the victim's femoral artery and she bleeds to death. I want the police to initially write this off as an accident. Would the murderer be covered with blood if she were standing behind the victim? How long would the victim take to die? How much blood would be around the victim?

Terri Thayer

A: A blade such as this could easily lacerate a femoral artery, which carries blood from the aorta to the leg. It lies near the surface in the groin, and its pulsations can be felt in the crease between the abdomen and the leg. This is a large artery, about the diameter of your thumb, and will bleed rapidly if severed. Less so if only nicked.

As with any severe arterial laceration, the victim would rapidly lose a great deal of blood (about two thirds of the blood volume, or approximately 4 to 5 pints). Initially it would come in spurts and gushes, then in weaker spurts, and finally in a steady flow. The reason is that as the blood is lost from the body, the blood pressure declines steadily so that the force pumping the blood from the artery falls almost beat by beat.

The time required for collapse and death depends upon many factors, such as the size and general health of the victim, the severity of the laceration of the artery, the position and activity of the victim after the injury, whether the victim knew what to do to stop the bleeding, and other factors. If the victim were young and healthy, if the artery were only nicked, and if the victim knew to apply pressure and call for help, she could survive, or it could take a half hour or more for her to exsanguinate (bleed to death). If the person was old and had heart disease, if the rip to the artery was large, and if the victim panicked and ran around, collapse and death could occur within five minutes or less. And anywhere in between. This means your timeline has very wide limits, and you can construct your scene almost any way you need. As your victim bled she would become weak, dizzy, cold, lethargic, maybe confused and disoriented, might shake and shiver, slip into shock, and die.

If the attacker were behind the victim she would likely avoid any blood, except on her hands. Of course, this blood will drip as she moves her hands away, and drops may fall behind the chair, where one would not expect to find them in a victim who remained in the chair until death. Crime-scene blood-spatter analysis would determine this, and this would create suspicion. How did the victim, if this truly was an accident, drip blood behind the chair? Or if the killer wiped her hands on the victim's clothing, this too might leave stains that the victim could not have made. Such findings might lead the ME to suspect murder rather than an accidental death.

If the victim fell from the chair to the floor, tried to reach a phone, or attempted to get to the door and call for help, blood-spatter analysis would reveal this. Based on the angle, direction, and length of the spurts, and the number and direction of any bloody footprints, drip and ooze spots, and other blood patterns, the analyst could determine the position of the victim at the time of the attack, and track any movements or change in position by the victim as she bled to death. All this is in the area of crime reconstruction, and some of the guys who do that are pretty good. You can use this to help your sleuth move the investigation in the right direction.

What Drug Could Cause a Stabbing Victim to Bleed More Profusely?

Q: In my story I have a victim who is stabbed. The killer has previously given him something that makes him bleed more freely. Is there a readily available drug that could do this? Would the ME be able to find the drug in the victim when he did an autopsy?

Michael Lister
Panama City, Florida
Author of the John Jordan mysteries
www.michaellister.com

A: Drugs that "thin" the blood are called anticoagulants. They will make someone prone to bleeding, particularly after an injury such as a stab wound. There are two that are easily available.

Coumadin (warfarin or coumarin) is a pill that must be taken over several days before it would have a significant anticoagulant effect. A single large dose might work, but even this would take a couple of days to have full effect. Why? It works by altering the liver's ability to construct certain proteins that are critical to blood clotting. Once the blood levels of these fall sufficiently, the person is more likely to bleed. This takes time. Your villain would need to surreptitiously add crushed Coumadin pills to the victim's food or drink for several days or a week before the stabbing.

Heparin is a liquid that must be given by either intravenous (IV) injection or by subcutaneous (sub q, or just beneath the skin) injection. The IV route is more effective and immediate. This can be given around the time of the stabbing, since it takes effect almost immediately. Your villain could stab the guy, subdue him, and inject the drug in a vein. The victim would then bleed profusely.

Blood normally clots in five to fifteen minutes after leaving the body. When the blood at the crime scene was found to be unclotted, the ME would know something was amiss. He would test the victim's blood and find that the results of the clotting tests were out of the normal range, and then do specialized testing to discover that either Coumadin or heparin was in the victim's body. If the victim had no reason to be on either of these medications, the possibility that it was given by another would be considered.

In a Death from Traumatic Injuries, Could My Killer Use CPR to Trick Investigators into Thinking the Death Was Due to a Gunshot Wound?

Q: Would it be possible to mimic circulation after death in order to obfuscate the cause of death? What I mean is, if the victim were to die from trauma caused by a car accident, but the suspect wanted it to appear as if the victim had been shot, would it be possible for the suspect to fire a bullet into the corpse of the victim, and then manually circulate the blood through the victim's system with CPR so that the wound would bleed, making it appear that the victim had been shot before he died?

A: The issues here are two: What exact traumatic injuries caused his death? What is the timing of the two events?

You are correct in assuming that a gunshot wound (GSW) in the living will bleed and one in a corpse will not. The dead don't bleed. At death the heart stops, the blood no longer circulates, and bleeding halts. So what you want is to move blood through the body after death so that a GSW will bleed a bit and make the ME believe that the GSW occurred premortem (before death).

Some traumatic injuries that occur in auto accidents can lead to immediate death. Things such as severe head injuries, decapitation, crush injuries to the chest or heart, penetrating injuries to the heart, brain, or major blood vessels, transection (cutting into two parts) or severe injury to the cervical (neck) spinal cord, and a few other things would fit this category. Other forms of injury lead to death from bleeding or from heart or lung compromise. In these situations the victim dies slowly, so that the exact time of death (stoppage of the heart) may not be seen easily.

If the victim had an injury to the heart or the major blood vessels, or if he bled a great deal before death, CPR would not move a lot of blood around. Maybe none. The reason is that, if most of the blood is on the street, there is little left to move. Also, if a major artery was sliced open or crushed, any blood movement that occurred from the CPR would preferentially take this path of least resistance and exit the body through this defect. You need an intact circulatory system if the CPR is to pump blood into the wound and cause blood collection in that area.

The time lag between the death and the gunshot wound (GSW) must be very short. Less than two minutes, for sure. Otherwise the blood would begin to clot, and that would be that. CPR will not move clotted blood.

But CPR may not be needed at all. If someone dies, and ten seconds later is shot, gravity will still cause liquid blood to seep into the tissues around the wound and, as it pools within the wound, some might leak out of it. Not much, but a little. It is very difficult for the ME to distinguish perimortem wounds (around the time of death) from truly postmortem wounds.

So your scenario would work if the victim was shot immediately after his accident and death. The sooner the better, with less than a minute being best. If he is shot more than two or so minutes later, the ME might be able to determine that the wound was postmortem. CPR may or may not extend that time to, say, three or four minutes, but it surely wouldn't extend it beyond that. So as long as you stay within these parameters your scenario should be believable.

Can My Killer Use a Paralytic Drug to Disguise as a Suicide a Murder in Which a Gun Was Used?

Q: My killer injects his victim with the paralytic drug suc-cinylcholine, puts a gun in the victim's hand (the killer is wearing rubber gloves), points the gun toward the victim's brain, and pulls the trigger. Will the ME know that this drug was administered? Would this show up on a test? I want them to find the drug, as it will be the main clue that reveals that this is a murder and not a suicide.

Ellin Pollachek, Ph.D.

A: The short answer is that, if they search diligently for sux (short for succinylcholine) they can find it. The trick is that they probably would not in the scenario that you describe. The ME would per-form an autopsy, and probably a routine drug and alcohol screen, neither of which would give any evidence that sux was involved.

So what would make the ME become suspicious and look fur-ther? Several things.

Maybe the victim had absolutely no reason to commit suicide but had enemies or people who might wish him harm. The family could raise questions, and the ME could order a forensic psychi-atric autopsy and discover that the victim was indeed not at high risk for suicide. A forensic psychiatric autopsy is the process of looking into all aspects of the victim's life, personality, and current stresses with an eye toward determining risk of suicide. If the results put him at very low risk, the ME would become suspicious.

Maybe there was a large insurance policy on his life and the insurance company refused to pay without a very thorough inves-tigation into the death. This is not uncommon.

The reconstruction of the crime scene might suggest that the gun was fired by another, thus eliminating suicide and raising the possibility of homicide. The nature of the entry wound can help determine the distance between the muzzle and the entry wound as well as the angle of the bullet's entry. If these are such that the victim could not possibly have held the weapon in that position, suicide is eliminated. If the blood-spatter pattern or the position of the victim and the gun were at odds with what would be expected in a self-inflicted gunshot wound, the ME would become suspicious. For example, finding the gun near the right hand of a lefty would raise questions, since people almost always shoot themselves using their dominant hand. And the gun essentially never lands in the shooter's lap in a suicide, yet killers often place it there.

Maybe during the autopsy the ME could find an out-of-the-way puncture wound, and he might begin to suspect that the victim had been injected by someone. This is particularly true if the injection site is somewhere where the victim could not easily have done it to himself. Behind the knee or in the creases where the buttocks join the legs are a couple of places where people try to hide injection marks.

If the ME was not suspicious and felt that the death was indeed a suicide, he would write it off as that, and that would be it. But if one of the above situations raised questions, he might dig deeper. He would perform toxicological tests on the victim's blood, urine, and stomach contents, and if he found an injection wound, on the tissues around the site. But keep in mind that thorough toxicological testing is expensive and time consuming, so he would not move down that path without good reason.

The tests he would use to find the sux would be the combination of gas chromatography and mass spectrometry (termed GC/MS for short). This combination of tests yields the "molecular fingerprint" for any chemical, and can thus identify any known chemical or compound. In the case of sux, both it and its breakdown products would likely be detectable.

Was It Possible to Uncover Laudanum in a Corpse in 1941?

Q: I am writing a mystery set in 1941 in which the victim dies of an overdose of laudanum. What would a medical examiner of that time have found when doing the autopsy to indicate that the poisoning had occurred?

A: Laudanum is a narcotic. Your victim would simply become drowsy, fall asleep, lapse into a coma, stop breathing, and die from asphyxia. Since there are no overt physical signs of laudanum (tincture of opium) poisoning, there would be no anatomical clues at autopsy. This is true of virtually all poisons, which means that finding them in a corpse requires chemical analysis.

Currently, we are able to uncover and determine the amount of virtually any toxin in a corpse. And the ME can use the level to estimate if the amount found was sufficient to cause, or at least to play a role in, the victim's death.

In 1941 the field of toxicology was in its infancy, but a chemist could detect arsenic, opiates and other plant alkaloids, and a few other substances. So your coroner may or may not be able to determine the cause of death. If he relied only on what he saw he would not, and he might say that the death was from natural causes. But if he took blood, urine, and tissue samples and sent them to a sophisticated (for that time) lab, he might be able to find the opiate and determine that its presence was related to the death. Or they could find nothing. The tests were not overly sensitive or reliable.

In 1941 the finding of any amount of the drug would be considered related to the cause of death. Unless the victim had been prescribed the drug by a physician or had purchased it in a pharmacy, that is. At that time, laudanum and paregoric (also tincture of opium) were commonly available, and were used for everything from headaches, insomnia, abdominal pains, and diarrhea to just about any other ailment you can think of. So if the victim had a legitimate reason to have the drug in his body, the coroner might deduce that this finding had nothing to do with the victim's death. Or he may conclude the opposite. He may even suggest that the death was a suicide. Any of these would be possible.

This gives you many ways to craft your story, depending upon what conclusion you want your ME to reach.

Can Toxicological Testing Distinguish Ativan from Restoril or Valium?

Q: A victim in my story is given Ativan in a drink and then knocked unconscious. He is then killed by carbon monoxide inhalation. I know the ME can use the combination of gas chromatography and mass spectrometry to find the drug, but can these tests distinguish Ativan from either Restoril or Valium? Two of my suspects take Ativan from time to time, so they would have access to it, but not the other two medications.

Nancy J. Sheedy
Frederick, Maryland

A: The toxicologist would have little difficulty identifying the exact drug.

The forensic toxicologist uses two general types of testing when looking for drugs in either a corpse or the living. Screening or presumptive tests determine what class the drug belongs to, and then confirmatory testing uncovers exactly which member of that class is present. The best confirmatory tests are the combination of gas chromatography (GC) and mass spectrometry (MS). Used together these are called GC/MS. Sometimes infrared spectrometry (IR) is used in conjunction with GC, and this combination is termed GC/IR. GC is used to separate compounds from one another, and sometimes the GC pattern alone might ID the drug. If not, MS or IR would be used to determine the exact chemical structure of each compound. MS and IR give a "chemical fingerprint" of any compound. They basically determine what elements are present and in what amounts, and this would give the chemical makeup of the compound in question. Every compound has a distinct chemical structure (this is what defines the compound, gives it its chemical name, and gives it its distinct properties), and thus an individual fingerprint.

Each of the drugs you mention is in the family of medications known as benzodiazepines. A routine drug screen of the victim's blood, urine, and/or liver tissue would show that the drug found belonged to this class. Since Ativan (lorazepam), Restoril (temazepam), and Valium (diazepam) would each appear on such screening tests, further testing with GC/MS would be needed to distinguish one from the other. By using these tests the ME could easily determine exactly which drug was present and in what amount.

Will Spraying Blood Products over a Bloody Crime Scene Obscure Luminol's Determination of the Original Blood Pattern?

Q: In the screenplay we're plotting a crew of expert cleaners is dispatched to remove all evidence of a gunshot murder. Instead of trying to clean all latent bloodstains, if they sprayed a dilute solution of blood or plasma over the area, would this interfere with Luminol's ability to define the original blood pattern?

A: Luminol reacts with minute traces of blood (down to parts per billion) and can determine the presence of blood even after extensive cleaning, and even after painting of the contaminated surfaces. It can show bleeding and spatter patterns, "trails" from a dragged body, or droplets from a fleeing perpetrator. Certain metals that are found in paints and other products, and certain chlorine cleaners, can obscure the results, since they also react with the Luminol. In the case of metals, the glow that results is very short-lived, compared to the glow from blood (which is also fairly short in duration), so an experienced criminalist may be able to tell the difference. Therefore, if your cleaning crew used a chlorine-type cleaner, this could hide the blood pattern. Of course, the ME could use other methods to determine the presence of blood, but the pattern might be obscured.

Yes, spraying blood would obscure the pattern and confuse the issue, since the Luminol would react equally with all the blood present. I would suggest you use blood and not plasma, since Luminol reacts with the hemoglobin molecule of the red blood cells (RBCs), which are abundant in blood. Plasma is the liquid part of the blood that remains after the cells are removed. No RBCs, no hemoglobin, no reaction. Spraying blood over the area would hide the spatter patterns, which are useful in crime-scene reconstruction. The criminalists would find an extensive amount of blood and take samples from the various surfaces. The ME might then be able to determine a DNA profile for the blood, and be able to determine that the blood was from two different sources—one from the victim and the other from an unknown source. He would likely interpret this as having come from two victims, and would not likely consider the scenario you propose. Clever.

Part IV

The Coroner, the Body, and the Autopsy

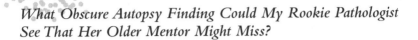

What Obscure Autopsy Finding Could My Rookie Pathologist See That Her Older Mentor Might Miss?

Q: The scenario: A young and marginally experienced pathologist is conducting an autopsy on a professional athlete in conjunction with her older and more experienced mentor. The athlete is known for his clean-cut, good-guy image. The tabloid speculation is that he died of some complication related to performance-enhancing drugs, but after the autopsy and before the tests come back, she determines he has died of something else that also goes against his image. Her mentor disagrees. I was thinking of an overdose of a recreational drug like crystal meth. Would this work?

Darwin Sauer
Victoria, British Columbia, Canada
Screenwriter of *The Barrens and Devil Monkey*

A: Either methamphetamine (crystal meth) or cocaine could work for your scenario. The young pathologist could have done her training in an inner-city hospital where she would see things that the old guy who worked in a more affluent area might not. One of these would be an autopsy on chronic snorters of meth or coke. This habit leads to scarring and ulceration (multiple tiny eroded areas) of the lining of the nasal passages. The tissues inside the nose are termed the nasal mucosa, and they are damaged by chronic cocaine or meth use. These drugs cause powerful constriction (narrowing or squeezing down) of the blood vessels in the nose, and this in turn leads to the death of the tissues, which will then ulcerate and scar.

Your rookie could have seen this many times while her mentor never had. This is common in all specialties of medicine. A physician might know what's in the books, but what he sees and has firsthand experience with depends upon the types of patients he actually sees. The older guy could be resistant to accept this possibility because of the victim's reputation. Only after the toxicology results came back, which could take several days, even weeks, depending upon the jurisdiction where your story occurs, would your heroine be proven correct.

How Long After Being Dumped into a River Will a Corpse No Longer Show Evidence of Molestation?

Q: I'm writing a book that takes place in the 1950s. A five-year-old male child has been molested, murdered, and thrown into a river. How long would it take for the corpse to deteriorate to the point that the coroners of that era could no longer determine that a sexual molestation had taken place?

A: Bodies dumped in water almost always sink. Then, as bacteria begin to grow and produce gas as one of the by-products of decay, the abdomen, chest cavity, and tissues fill with gas. This adds buoyancy, and the body rises to the surface. The time required depends upon the size and weight of the body and the rapidity with which the bacteria grow. The bacteria responsible for the internal gas formation come from within the body, the intestines predominantly. Bacteria in the environment may hasten decay, but since they attack the surface of the corpse they add little, if any, to the collection of internal gases.

A rule of thumb is that two weeks in the water equals one on land. Temperature determines the rapidity with which the bacteria grow and the gas forms. In this case it is the water temperature, and not the air temperature, that's important. The warmer the water, the faster the bacteria work. In the warm waters of the Gulf of Mexico, this process may take only a few days, whereas in a lake in the Canadian Rockies, it may take several months. An average lake or river in a temperate area would be somewhere in-between. A good range would be two to three weeks under most circumstances.

The body wouldn't likely be found until it floated, but it could of course be washed ashore by currents at any time, even while fairly well preserved. The sooner the body is found, the more well preserved it will be, and the more likely there would be evidence of assault. For the ME to see signs of sexual trauma or to find semen within the corpse, the corpse would need to be fairly intact. If it were significantly decayed, then his job would be more difficult, if not impossible.

It would be best if the body washed ashore a day or two after the assault, but even after three or four weeks, if the body is found shortly after it drifts to shore, there may still be evidence of sexual assault. Not necessarily, but possibly. The body could be so severely decayed that any evidence of trauma is no longer present.

If you want your ME to find evidence of the assault, have currents wash the body to shore after a couple of days, and have it discovered shortly thereafter. If you want to make sure that no evidence is left, have the body float to shore after a couple of weeks, and then lie there for another week or two. In this situation the body would be severely putrefied, and the ME would have little to work with.

The timeline for putrefaction varies greatly, so you can write your scene any way you wish within these broad parameters.

Is There a Formula for Accurately Determining the Time of Death from the Corpse's Body Temperature?

Q: While researching the timing of death for my story I ran across Marshall and Hoare's formula for estimating the time of death. Is this formula used? Accurate?

A: Marshall and Hoare's formula is rarely, if ever, used, since it is not accurate under most real-life situations. The reason is that it makes two basic assumptions that are fraught with inaccuracies. The first is that the body temperature at the time of death is "normal," whatever that is. Normal body temperature is stated to be 98.6 degrees Fahrenheit, but in fact this is not always the case. It varies from person to person, from circumstance to circumstance, and may even vary at different times of the day in a given individual. Second, it assumes that the ambient temperature is constant. This may be the case if a body is found in a room such as a basement or wine cellar, where the temperature varies very little, but this is rarely the case.

Inaccuracies in either of these assumptions can significantly alter the final estimation of time of death.

The most commonly used formula is also the simplest. Of course, it too is fraught with the same inaccuracies, but it doesn't require a computer to do it, as Marshall and Hoare's does. It is:

$$\text{hours since death} = \frac{98.6 - \text{body core temperature}}{1.5}$$

This means that, in general, under normal circumstances, a corpse loses heat at a rate of 1.5 degrees per hour. Using this scale, if a corpse is found to have a core temperature (usually either rectal or liver) of 92.5 degrees, death occurred approximately four hours earlier.

$$98.6 - 92.5 = 6.1$$

$$\frac{6.1}{1.5} = 4$$

This rule of thumb is about as accurate as anything else. It gives only an estimation of the time of death.

In a Death from Electrocution, What Are the Autopsy Findings?

Q: What internal and external signs can the coroner use to determine that a death was caused by electrocution?

Gina L. White
Los Angeles, California
Author of *The Corridor Murders*

A: Electricity comes in several flavors, and can kill by a couple of different mechanisms. Low-voltage currents are less than 600 to 1,000 volts, while high-voltage ones are in the range of 1,000 to 8,000 volts. Lightning is an extremely high voltage current. Virtually all deaths from electrical current are accidental, since it is rarely used for suicide or homicide.

When electricity enters the body it will flow from the point of entry to the point of grounding by following the shortest path. Whether the current is deadly depends upon its voltage and the duration of contact. A low-voltage current may take several minutes to do harm, while a high-voltage one may kill instantly.

Residential alternating current (AC) is low voltage and would cause only minor burns if the exposure is brief. With longer exposure time severe burns may result, and internal organs such as the liver and bone marrow may be severely and irreparably damaged. Death may follow.

The greatest danger of low-voltage shocks is their effect on the heart. The normal heartbeat is due to a rhythmic pulse of electrical current that originates in the heart's internal pacemaker and flows through the heart muscle. A low-voltage AC shock may interfere with this rhythmic pulse and lead to deadly cardiac arrhythmias (changes in heart rhythm) such as ventricular tachycardia and fibrillation. Death is typically instantaneous when this occurs.

High-voltage electrocutions occur in industrial settings and from the high-tension lines that carry current across the country and into neighborhoods. Local suburban and urban lines typically carry 700 to 8,000 volts, while the transcontinental lines carry 100,000 or more volts. Contact with these high-tension lines usually occurs when they fall to the ground in storms or accidents. Direct contact with such lines is not necessary, since the current may arc, or "jump," from the line to a person standing nearby. Also, any tall metallic object such as a ladder or a crane arm may carry the current to the victim. Such accidents are seen with the cherry-pickers used for tree trimming or TV cameras.

High-voltage AC shocks usually result in severe internal and external burning with even very brief exposures. But they are less likely to cause dangerous changes in the heart's rhythm. Why? Higher-voltage currents are defibrillatory rather than fibrillatory. This means that they convert an abnormal rhythm back to a normal rhythm rather than the other way around. In a cardiac arrest the external shock that physicians give to the victim is at a higher voltage. It is intended to restore a normal rhythm where a deadly, abnormal rhythm exists. However, high-voltage shocks may stop the heart completely, cause one of the above deadly cardiac rhythms, or paralyze the respiratory center in the brain, in which case death can follow from asphyxia.

At autopsy the ME will find several signs of electrical injury. In some low-, and all high-, voltage deaths, charred skin will be seen at the point of contact, the point of grounding, or both. Sometimes in low-voltage electrocutions there is no charring but rather redness and blistering at the contact point. In the case of a high-voltage arc there may be multiple small areas of burning, which represent the contact points of the arcing electricity. There may also be damage to some internal organs. The most commonly injured ones are the liver and the bone marrow.

One interesting phenomenon of electrocution deaths is the appearance of localized rigor mortis. The spasm of rigor mortis results when the adenosine triphosphate (ATP) in the muscles falls low after death. With electrocution the muscular spasm caused by the electrical current may consume the ATP and cause a more sudden onset of rigor in the affected area. For example, if someone grabs an electrical line with their right hand and the current passes down and out their right foot, their right arm and leg may show signs of rigor long before the rest of the body.

If the death was due to a low-voltage current, the ME may not be able to determine the exact cause of death. With higher-voltage currents the charring of the skin at the points of entry and exit, and the damage to the internal organs, would tell the story.

How Does the ME Determine What Weapon Caused a Particular Stab Wound?

Q: In my story the victim of a stab wound is found. How would the ME go about determining what weapon made the wound, and what would interfere with his ability to do so?

T. K. Harris
Huntsville, Alabama

A: Knives, scissors, axes, ice picks, and other sharp instruments cause penetrating or sharp-force injuries, as opposed to blunt-force injuries, which occur with baseball bats and metal pipes. Each of these sharp instruments causes different types of wounds.

Slashing, chopping, or cutting wounds are very difficult to analyze, but stab wounds might give the ME a great deal to work with. He will measure the depth and width of the wound and examine it for any unusual characteristics. The depth will give him the minimum length of the blade. It may be longer, but it can't be shorter than the depth of the wound.

Various weapons make various types of injuries. An ice pick will make a small, round wound that is fairly clean. A knife wound is longer and narrow. With a single-edged blade the width along the sharp edge will be narrower than that along the noncutting edge of the knife. This will not be seen with a double-edged knife. If the blade is curved, the ME may be able to determine the degree of curve. If the blade or the noncutting edge is serrated, he may find a roughened or abraded corresponding wound edge, which he would not see with a smooth-bladed weapon. If scissors were used, the wound characteristics depend upon how they were employed. If the blades are together, the wound will be wider than if the scissors were open and only one blade was used. If the blades are slightly apart, there will be two adjacent wounds, each of which will reflect the nature of the scissor blades.

If the ME is given a suspect weapon, he will carefully examine and measure its blade to see if its characteristics are consistent with his wound measurements. He will never actually insert the weapon into the wound, since this can alter the wound, which is evidence.

Even if the weapon and the wound are a perfect match, he can't say that this was the actual weapon used but rather only that it is similar. If he found the victim's blood on the blade or in the groove where the blade joined the handle, he could be more confident that this was the murder weapon. Or if the tip of the blade broke off in the wound he could analyze its composition and match that to the suspect broken-tipped knife. This would be an even stronger match. Better still, if the tip made a jigsaw match with the suspect blade, this would be very strong evidence that this was the murder weapon.

In evaluating fatal penetrating injuries the ME must also make several other determinations. With multiple injuries he must locate each and every wound, determine what type of weapon was likely used in each, and then estimate the sequence in which the wounds occurred. Finally, he must determine which wounds were potentially lethal. In homicides this becomes critical when there is more than one assailant, since the deliverer of the fatal wound could face the more serious charges. Sometimes these determinations are obvious, and other times not.

He must also determine the manner of death. Stabs, cuts, and chopping wounds can be accidental, suicidal, or homicidal in nature, and the ME must make this distinction whenever possible. He will use the nature, location, and number of wounds to make his evaluation.

What factors make the ME's task difficult or impossible? Sometimes the wound is clean, the corpse is intact, and the ME can learn a great deal about the weapon by examining the wound characteristics. At other times the wound is ragged, the corpse is partially decayed, the environment has changed the character of the wound, and the ME can obtain little useful knowledge from the wound. If the attacker twists or violently moves the weapon while it is imbedded in the wound, or if the victim turns or twists away from the attack, the wound may be severely altered and the ME would have little to work with.

Can the ME Distinguish Between an Ancient Skeleton and a Fresh One?

Q: How might an expert tell that a skeleton was one hundred years old rather than recent? The skeleton is of a young woman, a servant who was buried secretly in someone's backyard, no coffin or embalming. I want the police to be able to tell that this happened in the 1890s, and that she's not a recent murder victim.

A: The field of forensic anthropology is a fascinating but often inexact science. This is the case with dating skeletal remains. The bones can be used to determine the age, sex, size, and weight of the person, but determining the exact date of death is difficult. Yet the modern forensic anthropologist possesses several tools to aid him in this endeavor.

Every technique discussed here is greatly dependent upon the environment in which the victim was put to rest. In fact, the environmental conditions are more important than the elapsed time. For this reason great errors can be made in this estimation.

A skeleton found in a dry, cool area will be very different from one deposited in a warm, moist locale, even if both were buried at the same time. Those left in enclosed spaces such as crypts or rooms will be better preserved than those left to the elements and predators. Basically, the deterioration rate of the bones, cartilage, and soft tissues varies greatly, depending upon the conditions. A five-year-old skeleton left in the open may deteriorate as much as a hundred-year-old one left in a cool, dry crypt.

Bones are complex organs. They consist of a fibrous matrix

called "stroma" in which calcium and phosphorus are bound. They are *living* organs, which the body constantly tears down and rebuilds, and they serve as vast storage reservoirs for calcium and phosphorus, elements needed in many bodily functions. Bones that end in joints, like the elbow, hip, or knee, have cartilage at one or both ends and tendons and ligaments attached at various points along their length. Also, a thin layer of fibrous tissue called the periostium covers the bones.

The stroma, cartilage, periostium, tendons, and ligaments are considered soft tissue and are subject to deterioration, as are skin, muscle, and the internal organs. The rate of deterioration of these soft tissues is greatly affected by environmental conditions.

Recently buried bones will have all these soft-tissue remnants, while ancient ones will not. The periostium and tendon and ligament tags may survive five years or more. Of course, predators and adverse conditions could shorten this considerably.

If there are no soft-tissue remnants, the bones themselves may yield clues as to the timing of death. As the stroma deteriorates the bones become lighter, more brittle, and easier to cut. Very ancient bones may be brittle enough to flake or indent with a fingernail. This breakdown of the stroma occurs both outside-in and inside-out. That is, from the outer surface inward, and from the marrow cavity outward. This yields a "sandwich" effect. If a "fresh" bone is cut across the shaft, it will be hard and difficult to saw through. If an old one is similarly cut, the outer layer will cut easily, the middle area will be stronger and more resistant, and the inner layer will again cut more easily.

This sandwich effect is apparent if the cut end is viewed in a dark room under ultraviolet light. Here the fibrous stroma will fluoresce or glow a silvery blue tint. If this glow is seen to involve every layer, it means that the stroma has not begun to deteriorate and the bone is fresh. If the glow is confined to the middle section and is sandwiched between areas of no fluorescence, the bone is older. As time goes by and the stroma continues to decay, this fluorescent middle ring becomes narrower and narrower, until it finally disappears altogether. The time required for this process to become complete varies, but in general, complete loss of fluorescence requires 100 to 150 years. Your skeleton would be brittle, easily cut or flaked, and would show no fluorescence, or at most a very thin ring, in its middle portion.

Another test is the measurement of the amount of nitrogen (N) in the bones. N is found in the proteins that make up the stroma. As the stroma decays the level of N declines. Fresh bones are composed of approximately 4.5 percent N. If a bone contains more than 4 percent N, it is probably less than a hundred years old. If it contains less than 2.5 percent N, it is likely 350 or more years old. This test would be of little help for your detective.

Proteins are made of chains of amino acids (AAs). The proteins that comprise the stroma of bone contain fifteen different AAs. As the stroma deteriorates the amount of these AAs also declines. Two of these AAs, proline and hydroxyproline, disappear by about fifty years. The others may require hundreds of years to be undetectable. A bone with all the AAs is likely to be less than fifty years old, while those that contain only three or four AAs are likely to be hundreds of years old, as with your skeleton.

Radioactive isotopes help age bones. Carbon 14 (C-14) dating is of little use in forensics, since its ranges are too broad. The half-life (time it takes to decay by 50 percent) for C-14 is fifty-seven hundred years. It is useful for dating something that is many hundreds or thousands of years old, but not for those of shorter time periods. However, other radioactive materials may be helpful. With the testing and use of nuclear devices in World War II, and the continued testing throughout the 1950s and 1960s, the global environment saw an increase in C-14, strontium 90, cesium 137, and tritium (a radioisotope of hydrogen). Finding increased amounts of one or more of these in bones means that the victim died after about 1950. Those who died before this were not exposed to the environmental increase in these isotopes and would show no such elevation. The skeleton in your story would have none of these.

Can the Sex of a 150-Year-Old Skeleton Be Determined?

Q: What would the condition of human remains be after
being buried in a cellar for 150 years? Would broken
bones still be evident? Would my ME be able to tell if
the remains were male or female?

>   Heather Curley
>   Pittsburgh, Pennsylvania
>   curleyszone.blogspot.com

A: Depending upon the average ambient temperature, and the
general level of humidity in the area, the corpse would be either
skeletonized or mummified. Warmth and moisture favor putrefaction (decay), which would destroy all the tissues and leave behind
only bones. Cold and dry or hot and dry areas may allow mummification. Regardless, reduction to a skeleton is much more likely
than mummification.

After 150 years the bones could remain or not. In a protected
area such as you describe it is likely that at least some, if not all, of
them would still be present. And if the pelvis, skull, and jawbones
were present the sex of the person likely could be determined. If
all of these were missing, the task would be much more difficult, if
not impossible.

Determining the sex from skeletal remains of infants and children is more difficult than it is for adults. The reason for this is that
gender-specific changes in the skeleton do not appear until after
puberty. Between the ages of about twelve and twenty male and
female bones grow differently and begin to take on sex-identifying
characteristics. If the needed bones are available, the forensic anthropologist can use these variations to determine the sex of skeletal
remains.

The overall size and bone thickness of the male skeleton is
greater than that of the female. This is not universal, since bone
size and thickness is related to many things other than sex. Better
nutrition and heavy physical activity lead to stronger bones regard-

less of sex. So a female who ate well and performed manual labor might have a more male-appearing skeleton than a male who had poor nutrition and rarely worked physically.

Still, the thickness of certain areas of certain bones may be used to distinguish between males and females. In general the diameters of the heads of the humerus (upper arm bone), the radius (lower arm bone on the thumb side), and the femur (upper leg bone) are larger in males.

The most reliable bones used in sex determination are those of the pelvis. The male pelvis is designed only for support and movement, while the female pelvis is adapted for childbirth. The female pelvis is wider and possesses an increased diameter of the pelvic outlet, which allows the passage of the infant during childbirth. Also, the sciatic notch (where the sciatic and other nerves pass through on their way to the leg) is wider in females than in males. In addition, the backside of the pubic bone in women who have delivered a child may be scarred and irregular. This is due to the tearing and regrowth of ligaments that occur during childbirth.

The skull may also offer useful clues to the sex of the individual. Male skulls tend to have more distinct ridges and crests, and to be larger and thicker, particularly in areas where facial and jaw muscles attach. In addition, the posterior ramus of the mandible (jawbone) in males is slightly curved, while in females it tends to be straight.

As you can see, the ability to determine the sex of skeletal remains depends upon how many and which bones are present. If the skeleton is intact the accuracy is extremely high. If only a hip bone or a mandible is found, the job of the forensic anthropologist is more difficult, but he can still provide a fairly accurate guess. In the final analysis the only way to be absolutely certain is through DNA analysis, which in some cases can be extracted from bones and teeth. Not always, but sometimes.

How Would a Mummified Corpse Be Identified?

Q: My victim is now a mummified body. How long would it take to identify the mummified corpse of someone who has been dead about twenty-five years? I thought I could use the clothes to make the identification, but are there other ways I should consider?

Maureen Dowling
Port Jefferson, New York

A: The ME and the forensic anthropologist will use anything and everything at their disposal to identify and determine the cause and manner of death of any corpse, mummified or not, even one that has been deceased for several decades. And if a homicide is suspected, this identity takes on even more importance. Why? Because in the great majority of cases, perhaps 90 percent or more, people murder people they know. This means that identifying the victim will often narrow the suspect list and lead to the killer.

A mummy offers special challenges. The size, age, sex, and race of the victim would be determined easily in most cases, and this would narrow down the list of possibilities. If the victim was a forty-or-so-year-old male of about six feet in height, the ME would search missing persons' reports to see which ones might match that description. Clothing and other things found at the burial or dump site might also be critical. Of course, a wallet with a driver's license would help. Absent that, jewelry, belts, shoes, hats, and clothing are made and sold somewhere, and finding where they were manufactured and purchased might be critical in identifying the corpse. The type of plastic, tarp, or other material used to wrap the corpse might be identifiable, as would the materials used to make a casket, if one was used. Sometimes killers leave behind digging tools or other implements, even the murder weapon, and these might be helpful.

Tattoos and surgical scars may be visible. Tattoos are often so distinctive that they can be easily traced to the artist who did them. Surgical scars, such as those from open-heart surgery or a gallbladder removal, may serve to exclude some possibilities and include others. Surgical appliances such as hip replacements and pacemakers have serial numbers, making them very easy to track.

Fingerprints can sometimes be obtained from mummies by soaking the fingers in water or glycerin. This plumps them up, and prints can often be gotten that way. Or the skin of a finger can be sliced away carefully and pressed between two glass slides. A print may then become visible. These prints can be compared with those in a database such as the FBI's Automated Fingerprint Identification System (AFIS), or against the prints of those suspected of being the corpse. DNA and dental records may be compared to similar information available on any missing persons. After twenty-five years this may not be available, however.

The identification process can take a few minutes, a few hours, a few weeks, or forever. Many corpses are never identified. How long depends upon what is found and how quickly the police and ME can match that to a missing person. An example would be that the ME could obtain dental X-rays of the mummy. If the police had a missing person who had last been seen in the area of discovery and who matched the mummy in physical characteristics, he would have a forensic odontologist (dentist) compare those X-rays with the missing person's dental X-rays that he had obtained from their private dentist, and perhaps make an ID. This could take a few hours or a few days.

Is It Possible for the Coroner to Obtain DNA from a Forty-Year-Old Skeleton, and if So, Is It Useful for Identifying the Victim?

Q: The skeletal remains of a body that was buried in a canvas tarp forty years earlier is found. Would there still be hair with the remains? Would usable DNA be in the remains? If so, would strands of hair from forty years ago, retrieved for a keepsake lock of hair, yield follicles that would contain DNA that could be matched to the buried remains?

Jack Magccan
Richmond, Virginia

A: The overwhelming odds are that the corpse would be completely skeletonized after forty years. If the area was very hot and dry, it could mummify. If so, the ME would have dried tissues to work with, and DNA can sometimes be extracted from them. Not always, though. DNA could be present but be so damaged that it is of little use. In skeletons the bones and the pulp of the teeth might yield useful DNA. Or not. It can go either way. And if the keep-sake lock had follicles attached, DNA could be extracted from them and used to match DNA obtained from the bones or teeth. I should point out that if the lock were cut, there would be no folli-cles, but if it were pulled out, then maybe. But even if there are no follicles, all is not lost.

Hair may or may not be found at the burial site. You can have it either way. Hair itself contains no intact cells, and thus no nuclear DNA. Hair follicles do, but they would not be present in a skele-ton. Why? The follicle is made of hair-producing tissue, and this tissue would decay, as would the remainder of the body. Without follicular cells, standard DNA testing would not be possible. But mitochondrial DNA (mtDNA) can often be obtained from hair, and it can be useful for the identification of perpetrators and human remains, as well as for the determination of ancestry. Let me explain.

The DNA used for standard DNA testing is nuclear DNA. It can be extracted from any nucleated cell. But cells also contain nonnuclear DNA. This DNA is found within the mitochondria. Mitochondria are small organelles that reside within the cytoplasm of the cell (the soup) and serve as the cell's energy production cen-ter. A small amount of DNA is found within the mitochondria, but each cell has many mitochondria organelles. So why is mitochon-drial DNA important? Several reasons.

Mitochondrial DNA is passed from generation to generation through the maternal lineage, mutates rarely, is found in places where nuclear DNA doesn't exist, and is exceptionally hardy.

Your mtDNA is inherited unchanged from your mother, and only from your mother. And she received hers from her mother, and her mother from her mother, and so on. Why is this? At fertil-ization the egg supplies the cell and half the DNA, while the sperm supplies only half the DNA. This means that all the cell compo-nents of the developing zygote, including the mitochondria, come from the mother. As the cell divides and multiplies, these mitochondria are copied and passed on, generation after generation. This means that all the cells of the body contain identical mtDNA.

Also, mtDNA rarely mutates. It is thought to undergo a significant mutation approximately once every sixty-five hundred years, which means that your mtDNA is identical to your mother's, your great-great-grandmother's, and your maternal ancestors' from a thousand years ago. Thus, your maternal lineage can be traced accurately over many generations.

Since hair is composed of dead follicle cells that have lost their nuclei, it contains mtDNA but not nuclear DNA. So if you had a suspected descendant of the corpse, and the descendant's maternal ancestry appeared to lead back to the corpse, the mtDNA could prove that the corpse and the suspected descendant were indeed related down the maternal line. This may be very useful in identifying the skeletal corpse.

If the mtDNA in the lock of hair matched the mtDNA of hair found at the burial site, it would mean that the skeleton could be the person in question, or could be someone maternally related to the person from whom the lock of hair was taken. Most often this is enough to establish identity.

Do Twins Have the Same DNA Profile?

Q: In my story the existence of a twin is unknown. A rape and murder has been committed and a suspect apprehended. Would there be a difference in the DNA if the suspect's twin had committed the crime?

Paul Boucher
Perth, Australia

A: It depends upon whether the two were identical or fraternal twins.

Typically at conception, one sperm mates with one egg. This produces a zygote that will grow by repetitive cell division until an embryo results. The embryo continues to develop into a fetus, and ultimately a child.

If two sperm mate with two eggs, twins will result. The union of sperm A and egg A would produce child A, while the union of sperm B and egg B would yield child B. These would be two distinct individuals with their own special DNA profiles. They would be as different as if they had been conceived at different times. They are twins simply because they share the mother's womb at the same time. These would be fraternal twins, and each would have his own unique DNA.

On the other hand, if sperm A mates with egg A to make child A as usual, but when the first cell division takes place the two daughter cells separate, then two A children will result. Neither sperm B nor egg B is involved here. Each zygote would contain the DNA from sperm A and egg A, and each would continue to divide and grow into a fetus. But since they both came from the same egg and sperm, they would have identical DNA. These would be identical twins.

In your scenario, if the two were fraternal twins the DNA from each would not match, but if they were identical twins, the DNA profile of each would be the same. However, even identical twins have different fingerprints. I have no idea why this is the case, but it is.

By Using DNA Analysis, How Long Does It Take to Determine That a Rape Has Occurred?

Q: If a woman dies of multiple stab wounds and her body is recovered within a couple of hours of her death, how long does it take to determine whether she was raped? How long to analyze the DNA of the semen?

Glenn Ickler

Hopedale, Massachusetts

Author of *Camping on Deadly Grounds* and *Stage Fright*

A: First of all, rape is not a medical term, so the ME who examined the body cannot state whether a rape occurred or not. Rape is a legal term, and it can only be determined by a judge or jury. What the ME can determine is whether there is any evidence of forceful injury, penetration, and intercourse. If he can show these things, then the jury can use this information to determine if the sexual penetration was consensual or forced. Another important determination the ME can make is an estimate of the time since intercourse. This can be used to corroborate or refute victim, witness, and/or suspect statements and alibis.

Rape is rarely about sex, but rather is more about violence, control, and possibly humiliation. In order for rape to be charged, three things must have occurred: actual penetration; the use of force; and the lack of consent. Penetration does not need to be complete; only slight penetration is needed to meet the definition of rape. Force may be applied through violence, the threat of violence, or coercion, including the use of drugs for this purpose. All too often rape is accompanied by homicide, either as part of the violent act or following it to prevent the victim from identifying the assailant. Rape is often part of the act of homicide by a serial killer, particularly the sexually sadistic types. In this case the rape is almost always part of the killer's fantasy, or of his need to humiliate the victim.

In a living rape victim it is critical that a complete rape exam be done as soon after the act as possible. Unfortunately, because the act is so humiliating for the victim, she will often wait days, if not months or years, before reporting it. At other times the victim will shower or bathe before going to authorities or to a hospital. On the surface this may seem to be odd behavior for an assault victim, but rape is not like a punch in the face. It carries with it an array of emotions and social baggage that no other crime does. Often the victim feels ashamed, even guilty, and for sure wants to avoid the inappropriate but real feeling of social stigmatization. Remnants of puritanical thinking and a court system that all too often makes the victim feel as though she is on trial play a role in these feelings.

A medical doctor experienced in rape examinations should examine the living victim. If possible, a law enforcement officer should be present so that the chain of evidence can be maintained. The examination consists of obtaining a medical history, performing a complete physical exam, taking photographs if indicated, and collecting evidence. Of course, the treatment of any serious or life-threatening injuries to the victim takes precedence over evidence collection.

The physician will examine the victim's entire body, including the genitalia, for evidence of trauma such as bruises, abrasions, or lacerations. He will carefully note and photograph each. It is important to note that the absence of signs of trauma or violence in no way negates or diminishes the claim that a rape has occurred. Any bite marks will be photographed and swabbed for saliva, which may yield DNA. Any stains will likewise be swabbed, since they could represent saliva or semen. As guided by the history the victim gives as to what transpired during the assault, the examining physician will obtain vaginal, anal, and oral swabs for DNA-containing materials. The victim's pubic hair will be combed for foreign hairs and fibers. Last, the victim's clothing will be examined for stains, and if any are found, samples will be taken and the clothing packaged and taken to the crime lab for evaluation. Indeed, all evidence collected is turned over to law enforcement for transport to the crime lab for study.

Once the examination is completed, the victim's injures are treated and she is given medications to prevent pregnancy and to treat any possible venereal disease. A wait-and-see attitude is not adopted in this situation, but rather the philosophy is to treat these possibilities soon. A blood sample for HIV testing is obtained, and will be repeated over the next several months. A rape counselor usually becomes involved immediately to help the victim with the psychological fallout from the assault.

In rape-homicides, as is the case in your scenario, many of the same examinations are taken, except that a history of the events is typically absent and the ME rather than a physician performs the examination. As with any homicide it is best if the ME sees the body at the crime scene, but for practical reasons this is not always possible. At the scene the coroner's investigators are charged with transporting the body and protecting the evidence. Paper bags are secured over the victim's hands, and the body is placed in a clean body bag or wrapped in clean sheets for transport. This prevents the loss of trace evidence and lessens the likelihood that the corpse will pick up any trace materials during transport.

At the lab the ME initially will examine the victim while clothed. He will look for any trace evidence and stains, and attempt to match any defects in the clothing with injuries to the victim. Only then will the clothes be removed and sent to the crime lab for further processing. After this he will turn his attention to the body.

The body will be searched for foreign hair, fibers, or other trace evidence. Stains will be examined and swabbed. After the protective bags over the victim's hands have been removed, the ME will carefully examine the hands and collect nail clippings and scrapings. Often the assailant's hair, blood, or skin tissues may be found clutched in the victim's hand or beneath her fingernails. All injuries, including those to the genitalia, will be examined and photographed. A diligent search for evidence of penetration will follow, and vaginal, anal, and oral swabs will be obtained.

Even if no overt trauma is found, the ME will look for signs that sexual intercourse took place. Vaginal fluids will be examined for evidence of semen. This will be done chemically and microscopically. Tests for acid phosphatase, an enzyme found in abundant quantities in semen, and P30, a semen-specific glycoprotein, will be done. Acid phosphatase may be present up to seventy-two hours after intercourse. A problem arises when the victim has had consensual sex during the two or three days before the assault. There is no method for determining if elevated levels of acid phosphatase are remnants of this consensual act or of the rape itself.

A search for spermatozoa will also be undertaken. In living victims motile sperm may be seen up to about twelve hours after intercourse, and rarely, up to twenty-four hours. Nonmotile sperm may persist for two or three days. As sperm die off they initially lose their tails, leaving behind only sperm heads. These may be seen up to seven days after intercourse. So if the victim states that she last had consensual intercourse three days earlier, the finding of nonmotile sperm or sperm heads is of little help, but any motile sperm could not have come from that episode and must be related to the rape.

Sperm lasts longer in a corpse than in a living victim. The reason is that in the living the vagina produces certain chemicals that destroy sperm, while in a corpse sperm are destroyed only through decomposition, which requires many days. Sperm can be found for up to two weeks in a corpse.

Even if no sperm are found, intercourse cannot be ruled out. The assailant may have used a condom, had a previous vasectomy, failed to ejaculate, or been azoospermic. Azoospermia is a condition in which no sperm is produced.

The time required depends upon how quickly the autopsy is done. If rushed, it could be done the same day that the body was found, and if not would be done usually within twenty-four to forty-eight hours. This varies from jurisdiction to jurisdiction, depending upon the ME's workload, his budget, the number of pathologists available for the work, and other factors. During the autopsy the ME could likely determine if trauma or penetration occurred, and the following microscopic examination of the vaginal swabs would reveal if sperm were present, thus proving that intercourse with ejaculation occurred.

DNA analysis could be done in twenty-four hours, and the ME might then give the police a preliminary verbal report if this could help their investigation. However, his official report would take several days, if not weeks. Why? It's his reputation on the line, and he would double-check his results before filing a final report. A mistake at that point could jeopardize the entire case. So he would send samples to one or more DNA testing labs and await their independent determinations. If the two or three labs involved all gave the same result, he could finalize his report with confidence.

In a Death Caused by a Beating, Can the Coroner Distinguish Injuries Inflicted by Fists from Those by a Stick?

Q: In examining a corpse where a boxer is the likely assailant, would the coroner be likely to notice that the man was beaten to death with fists and a wooden handle, or would he likely think only fists were used? This takes place in 1948, if that makes a difference.

Warren Bull
Author of *Abraham Lincoln for the Defense*
www.warrenbull.com

A: Maybe. The coroner would examine the body and the wounds. He might see bruises that were long and thin and looked as though they had been made by a stick or handle. If he had the suspected murder weapon he might be able to match the shape of the weapon to some of the bruises on the victim. And if the handle bore some sort of pattern, the bruises might reflect this pattern. This latter detail would be very strong evidence.

If the handle were wooden or painted, or both, he might find splinters or flecks of paint that would not only match the wood or paint but might even match the missing pieces on the weapon, like pieces of a jigsaw puzzle. Such a match is highly specific and very strong evidence. For example, if he found a paint fleck in the victim's skin or scalp and could match it exactly to a fleck missing from the suspect weapon, this would be very damning evidence. What are the odds that two pieces from two different sources would match in such a manner? Very remote. So such a match would prove that the weapon was indeed the source of the paint fleck found on the victim. The only special equipment he would need to make this comparison would be a magnifying glass or a microscope.

What Happens to the Fetus if the Pregnant Mother Is Murdered and Dumped in a Lake?

Q: My story involves the murder of a pregnant woman. My question concerns what happens to a thirty-three-week-old fetus after the mother is murdered and dumped into a lake. The body washes ashore after about three months. Will the fetus decay along with the mother, or would it be relatively protected?

A: Either is possible, but most likely the fetus would be relatively protected. What happens and how quickly it happens depends upon the water temperature, the action of any marine predators, and any trauma the corpse might suffer from currents, boats, and other objects.

A body will initially sink when it is thrown into a body of water. As the putrefaction process takes place the bacteria that cause this decay produce gas, which collects within the body's cavities and tissues. When enough gas collects the body will rise to the surface. We call these "floaters." How quickly a body will float depends upon how rapidly the gas collects, which in turn depends upon how active the bacteria are. Bacteria thrive in warmth and are greatly slowed by cold. So a corpse tossed into a Louisiana swamp may float in a day or two, while one placed in a lake in Minnesota may not rise for many months.

This is what happens to the mother, but what about the fetus?

The fetus is relatively protected so long as it remains within the uterus. As the mother decays, gases will accumulate within the mother's abdomen. As this process continues, the pressure will rise, the belly will distend, and the fetus might be forced from the uterus through the birth canal and out of the mother. This is called a "coffin birth."

This is what happened in the famous case of Laci Peterson's murder by her husband, Scott. The pregnant Laci was murdered and dumped into San Francisco Bay. Nearly four months later Laci and her unborn son, Conner, washed ashore. Laci's body was severely decayed, while baby Conner's was relatively intact. This would suggest that Conner remained within his mother until shortly before the bodies were found. The cold water slowed the decay process so that three to four months were needed before enough gas built up to cause the mother's body to float and the coffin birth to occur.

So what happens in your scenario depends upon the water temperature. If warm, the process may take only a few days to a couple of weeks, and the fetus would be more decayed. In colder water the process may take several months, and the fetus could be relatively intact.

In a Death Due to Wrist Slashing, Can the ME Distinguish Murder from Suicide?

Q: What evidence does the ME use to distinguish murder from suicide in the case of a person with slashed wrists?

A: He may or may not be able to distinguish between the two. But the things he would look for would be:

> **The angle of the cuts:** Could the person have held a knife and made cuts at that angle? The blade would cut the wrist differently depending on whether the victim or the murderer held it. For example, if the cut went from the little finger (ulnar) side to the thumb (radial) side, this would be awkward for someone to do to himself. It could be done, but if the ME saw it he would be suspicious. The logical way would be just the opposite—the wrist laid flat in the lap or on the bed or the side of the tub, and the cut following a radial to ulnar direction.

> **Hesitation marks:** People attempting suicide almost always make a couple of weak cuts before cutting deeply enough to sever an artery. Why? First of all, it hurts like hell. Also, the cut needs to be much deeper and requires more force than most people imagine. Thus, there would be several shallow cuts, nicks, and scratches before the victim gathered the courage to cut deeply. Most people stop with the shallow cuts. It's just too painful and not as theatrical as they had envisioned.

> **The bleeding pattern:** Blood follows gravity and flows downhill. If the victim is sitting, the blood would drip and flow over his lap, legs, shoes, and the floor. If he is lying down, the blood would flow onto the bed. If the bleeding pattern doesn't match the location and position of the victim, the ME might become suspicious.

The nature of the cuts: If both wrists were cut the ME would make sure the victim could actually have done that. To cut the arteries in the wrist, the slice would also likely cut the tendons to the hand and fingers. This means the fingers and hand wouldn't work too well anymore. This isn't always the case, but if it is, it's not likely a suicide. If the tendons were cut, the victim would not be able to grasp a knife, and thus could not have cut the other wrist.

The weapon: The victim's fingerprints should be on the weapon, and they should be in locations one would expect if he had held the knife. If not, the ME would worry and dig further. If the weapon had disappeared from the scene, that would point toward homicide. Suicide victims don't usually get rid of the weapon. Or, if they do, leave a blood trail to wherever they toss it.

A psychological autopsy: People commit suicide for a reason. A forensic psychiatrist would delve into the victim's history, including family, work, social situations, drug habits, and other things. If he found a happy person with big future plans and stable relationships, he would wonder if this were the type of person who would commit suicide. If the victim was depressed, had just had a breakup or lost a job, or had some awful illness, then suicide becomes more likely. And the absence of a suicide note or some similar communication with a loved one is always bothersome. Not that one is always left, but it is common.

Can an Autopsy Reveal That My Character Has Had a Major Facial Reconstruction?

Q: My ME examined the mangled corpse of a man who was attacked by a shark. He learned that the victim, who was a fugitive from the law, had had major reconstructive surgery to change his appearance. Could he determine this during an autopsy? And is it possible that a forensic artist could "deconstruct" the changes and determine what the victim looked like before the plastic surgery?

A: Great question.

Plastic techniques leave very small scars, but they are scars nonetheless. The ME could see these if he looked closely enough. Usually the scars are around the eyes, at the temples, the ears, and the forehead in the case of a face-lift, and in the creases at either side of the nose and within the nose in a rhinoplasty (nose job). If the bones and cartilage of the nose had been hammered and chiseled, he would see evidence for this in the form of scars. Bone scars are called caliuses. If implants or bone grafts were placed to build up the cheeks or chin, these would be readily apparent. Since facial plastic surgery often employs all these techniques, the ME would likely have no problem determining that the victim had undergone a reconstructive procedure.

As to whether it is possible for a forensic artist to turn back the clock and re-create the victim's original appearance, I will say that these artists are very good. Some use drawings and others use three-dimensional models. In either case it would be a "best guess." But based on the unaltered facial features and the general shape of the head, face, and jaw, the artist could "reconstruct" a good guess, and it would likely be close, if not exact.

Could a Death from Smothering or Strangulation Be Made to Look Like a Suicidal Jump from a Tall Building?

Q: I have a victim who is strangled or smothered and the body is placed at the foot of a tall building to look as if she'd jumped. What would be the giveaway marks/bruising/clues as to the truth, and how long after death would such marks appear?

Rosemary Lord

Los Angeles, California

Author of *Hollywood Then and Now* and *Los Angeles Then and Now*

A: There are several signs that strangulation or smothering has occurred, and these could tip off the ME as to what actually caused the death. Or they may not be present and he may not be able to say.

Smothering occurs when some external device prevents air from entering the nose or mouth. This is distinguished from choking, in which the obstructing material is *within* the mouth or throat. Homicidal smothering usually employs a pillow, bedding, plastic bag, or the killer's hands. When a pillow or a plastic bag is used, marks on the victim typically are not present unless the victim puts up a struggle. If so, abrasions or bruises are often left on the victim's face or arms by the killer's attempts to control the victim. If there are no external bruises, and if the pillow or bag is removed before the body is found, the ME may not be able to determine the cause of death, since smothering itself leaves behind little physical evidence.

When a killer uses strangulation as a method of murder, typically either a ligature or his hands are used. If by hand it is termed manual strangulation. If by a rope, cord, wire, or other flexible material, it is called ligature strangulation. Hanging is basically strangulation in which the body weight is used to tighten the ligature, which is most often a rope. Manual and ligature strangulation are almost always homicide, while hangings are predominately suicide.

The cause of death in all strangulations is cerebral hypoxia, which is a low level of oxygen in the brain. This results because strangulation blocks the airway, preventing the victim from breathing, and occludes the carotid arteries, thus preventing the flow of blood to the brain. Of these two, the occlusion of the arteries is the predominant cause of unconsciousness and death. The carotid arteries pass from the aorta to the brain by way of the neck, and are the major sources of blood supply to the brain.

A common, though not universal, finding in all types of strangulation is petechial hemorrhages in the conjunctivae (the pink parts around the eyeball) and the sclera (the white part) of the eyes. Petechial hemorrhages (or petechiae) are small red dots or streaks that are due to blood leaking into the soft conjunctivae and sclera of the eyes. With strangulation, the pressures within the veins of the neck rise suddenly and dramatically. This pressure is transmitted to the veins of the eyes, causing them to leak blood and produce the petechial hemorrhages.

The marks found on the victim's neck are often a combination of contusions (bruises) and abrasions (scrapes). The pressure from the assailant's fingers in manual strangulations may leave bruises in the shapes of fingers. Abrasions may result from the assailant's fingernails. Since the tips of the fingers are used to grip the victim's neck, the attacker's nails may dig into or scratch the victim's flesh.

In manual strangulation, the victim's face is typically congested, and petechial hemorrhages are commonly seen. Since most assailants use a great deal more force than is necessary, there may also be injury to the neck muscles, and the ME will often find bleeding into these muscles at autopsy. Also, the small bones of the neck are often injured. Fractures of the cornu (horn) of the thyroid cartilage (Adam's apple) and the tiny hyoid bone are the norm in manual assaults.

Ligature strangulation occurs when a constricting band is tightened around the neck. Devices typically used are ropes, wires, electrical cords, and clothing such as neckties, belts, and stockings. If the device is soft, such as a towel or bedsheet, no marks may be visible on the neck, because the bruising left behind might be broad, diffuse, and not easily seen. In fact, if the soft ligature is removed from the victim, the ME will have a more difficult time in determining the exact cause of death. If the ligature is thin, such as an electrical cord, a deep groove or furrow will remain in the tissue of the victim's neck. Occasionally the bruises will reveal the pattern of the ligature used. The braids of a rope or the links of a chain may be readily visible.

In ligature strangulation, as with the manual variety, the victim's face is typically congested, and scleral and conjunctival petechiae are seen. However, in contrast to manual strangulation, bleeding into the neck muscles and fractures of the thyroid cartilage and the hyoid bone are much less common.

If the ME found signs of strangulation or smothering, he could determine that this was the cause of death. If none of these signs were present (pillow or plastic bag suffocations would be best for this) he might not be able to say this.

The problem with your scenario is the placing of the body on the ground. Here there would be no fall-related injuries, so the ME would not conclude that a fall was the cause of death. If the victim had no traumatic injuries he would rightly conclude that the body was either killed or placed at the spot where it was found. Falls kill by damaging brains, organs, and bones. Depending on the distance, a fall could lead to very few injuries or to very severe ones, such as broken bones and ruptured internal organs. In the absence of such findings the ME would never conclude that the victim died from a fall.

So your bad guys should toss the victim off the building so that these injuries would be present. If so, the problem would then be one of timing. If the victim was smothered and tossed off the building immediately the injuries would show signs of bleeding. For example, if the femur (the large bone of the upper leg) fractured there would be bleeding around the fracture. Here, if there were no signs of strangulation, and there was bleeding around broken bones and a ruptured spleen and kidneys, the ME might write off the death as a fall, which could be either an accident, a suicide, or a homicide. That would require police work to determine.

But if more than three or four minutes passed between the strangulation and the fall, there would be no bleeding. Why? The dead don't bleed. At death the heart stops, the blood ceases to circulate, and the blood clots in a very few minutes. If the ME found fractures and ruptured organs with no bleeding he would know that the injuries had occurred after death, and since dead people not only don't bleed but also can't jump from buildings, he would know he was dealing with a homicide.

During an Autopsy, Can the Coroner Distinguish Bruises from an Assault from Those Suffered from a Fall?

Q: In my story the victim gets beaten up and then falls off a rocky ocean cliff. He is found washed ashore, less than twelve hours later. Will the ME be able to distinguish those bruises and scrapes gotten from the rocks from the ones sustained from the perpetrator? Also, if my victim was punched hard enough, is it possible to find impression marks left by the attacker's ring on his face, or would being in the water destroy any impression?

Lyn Tucker

Carlsbad, California

A: From your question, I'm assuming that your victim was beaten but alive when he went off the cliff. If so, under most circumstances the ME would not be able to distinguish bruises and abrasions that occurred with the beating from those that happened with the fall. There are several exceptions, however, that should be useful to you.

If the victim received penetrating wounds from a knife or ice pick or another sharp object, the wounds might be so distinctive that the ME would conclude that they could not have come from falling on rocks or branches or whatever. If a suspect weapon were found he could measure and compare the wounds as to length, width, and depth, and say that the weapon in question was consistent with the wounds. Or not. It could go either way.

Blunt-force trauma as from a fist, stick, or fall would cause bruising if the injuries occurred while the victim was alive, or in the very immediate postmortem period, say a minute or two. Postmortem injuries do not bruise. So if the victim were alive when he was tossed or fell, the bruises he incurred would be a combination of those he received during the beating and those that occurred from the fall.

Occasionally a bruise may mimic the pattern of the object that made it. If your victim had been held or restrained during the beating, he might show bruises on his arms, and these bruises could reflect a finger pattern. If he had been tied with a rope or some other material, he might have bruises on his skin, and these might reveal the width and even the weave pattern of the rope. Or if he were beaten with a chain or a board, the bruises could reveal the links of the chain or the parallel edges of the board. And if your killer wore a distinctive ring with a large logo, design, or initial on it, it is possible that the bruise would mimic this design.

Since bruises are caused by bleeding into the skin and lie beneath the skin's surface, the water would have little effect on them until putrefaction set in and the bruised tissues were destroyed. In cool water this decay process could take two weeks or more, so this isn't an issue for your scenario.

What Would a Corpse Look Like After Two Months on a Cold Mountain?

Q: In my story a body has been lying unprotected for two months (April and May) above the frost line in the White Mountains of northern New Hampshire when it is discovered. It was frozen for the month of April and alternately freezing and thawing during the month of May. I imagine this would retard the standard rate of decay. I would like to know if there would still be any tissue left, or would the remains be skeletal, and would the corpse have an odor?

A: In your scenario the consistently below freezing weather for April would prevent any significant decay of the body. As the weather warmed periodically in May the body would begin to thaw, and this would allow for some bacterial growth, and thus decay. This would be a slow process, since the temperature would never reach what could be considered warm. This means that the decay would be slow, and even after four weeks the body would not be severely putrefied. So yes, your corpse would still have a significant amount of tissue, and most, if not all, of the internal organs intact. The ME would then have DNA, dental patterns, and likely even fingerprints to work with.

Another point of interest would be that the body would decay outside-in. Under normal circumstances and temperate conditions, a body will decay from the inside out. The reason is that the bacteria responsible for putrefaction come predominantly from the victim's intestinal tract and not from the environment. Thus, the internal organs begin the decay process first. But with a frozen corpse the thawing would occur over the surface, while the inside would remain frozen. Each day, when the temperature rose above freezing, the first inch or so of tissue would thaw, bacterial growth, though slow, would begin, and the decay process would be initiated. Each night this outside layer would again freeze. The next day the thawing would occur once again, the bacteria would resume their activity, and a little more decay would result. Day by day this process would repeat itself. The internal organs would not thaw, so the bacteria in the intestinal tract would never really get a chance to go to work. Thus, the body would decay from the outside in. How fast this decay actually occurred would depend upon many things, but the most important would be exactly how high the daytime temperature was, and how long it was at that level.

One of the questions the ME wants to answer is, when did the person die? Was it two weeks ago, or two months ago? This timeline might be critical to identifying a suspect and obtaining a verdict. The ME might consult with a forensic climatologist, who would review weather charts and attempt to determine the pattern of temperature changes around the location of the corpse. This may help in the determination of how long the body must have been there to decay to the degree found. It would be a crude guess but could narrow the time frame down to a week or so, and this might be helpful in solving the crime. This is an inexact science, and the ME could only make his best guess.

Since some degree of the decay process would be ongoing, there would be an odor of decay surrounding the body. It may be faint and require someone to be fairly close to the corpse to detect it.

Can the ME Determine Where a Drowning Took Place by Examining the Water in the Victim's Lungs?

Q: In a drowning victim, if there is air in the lungs, does the body float faceup? If not, what determines the position of body? How accurately can the ME determine the source of the water? That is, can he determine that the drowning occurred in a bathtub rather than a creek, or a creek as opposed to a lake?

Jack Chalfin

Dennis, Massachusetts

Author of *Memoirs of a Moth*

A: Air in the lungs has little or nothing to do with whether a body floats faceup or facedown. In fact, all bodies sink first, and then float only after several days or weeks or months (depending on the water temperature), when the decay process produces gases that collect in the body's cavities and tissues. The body can then float in any position, though usually facedown.

Often the ME can test the water that is found in a drowning victim's lungs and stomach (drowning victims often swallow a great deal of water in the struggle for survival) and determine the water type and, occasionally, its location. Salt water, fresh water, and pool water can most often be distinguished from one another, though not always.

Since a drowning victim inhales bits of debris, plant life, and animal life along with the water, the site of the drowning may be located. For example, in a freshwater drowning, if the lungs contain bits of leaves, seeds, or pollen from a plant that only grows in a particular pond or lake, the ME might say that the drowning likely took place in that pond or lake. The same can be said for certain types of tiny animal life that are found in one body of water but not in another. Pool water might contain chlorine, and bath water might contain soap or oils, and these can sometimes be identified. The fresh-water versus salt-water drowning scenario was used to great effect in the movie *Chinatown*.

Can the ME Determine That My Victim Drowned in a Punch Bowl and Not in a Lake?

Q: In my story the cause of a young woman's death is drowning. Her car is found near a lake. Actually, she died when the killer held her head in a punch bowl. Would there be traces of sugar and alcohol in her lungs if she drowned in spiked punch? Could the ME figure that out?

> Erica Printz
> Van Nuys, California

A: Maybe yes, maybe no. It can go either way. Most likely the ME would find colored fluid in her lungs and stomach and would analyze it. The high sugar and alcohol level would suggest punch or some other fruity liquid. If the liquid was found within her bronchi (breathing tubes) and lungs, he might conclude that she drowned in this liquid and not in the lake. Also, in most open-water drownings, visible and microscopic plant and animal life and debris can be found in the lungs. As the person inhales the water, he also inhales all the tiny things in the water. Leaves, bugs, and microscopic creatures can often be found. These things aren't usually present in a punch bowl. And if the victim were dead at the time she went into the lake, she would not inhale any of the bug-and-debris-containing water, so none would be found.

If the ME found a colored sugar- and alcohol-containing liquid, and not water and debris, in her lungs he might conclude that the victim was drowned in a bowl of punch and dumped in the lake. Or he might find none of this and might not be able to say where the victim drowned. In your story you can have it either way and it'll work.

Can a Death Blow to the Head Be Masked by a Gunshot Through the Same Wound, Thus Making the Death Appear to Be a Suicide?

Q: Here's what I've imagined: My two characters get into a fight. In the heat of the moment, one pushes the other, who falls and hits his head on the corner of a glass table and either is killed from the blow or appears to be dead. The pusher panics and decides to cover this up by disguising it as a suicide. He places the handgun into the victim's hand, presses it against his head, and shoots. Could the gunshot really cover up the initial blow to the head?

Roberta Isleib
Author of the Advice Column mysteries
www.robertaisleib.com

A: It's possible. If he fired the gun through the wound, the entry wound would likely be small and the ME would see the other trauma. There would be a small, round entry wound in the middle of an area of contusion (bruising). It would be better to fire from the other side of the head and have the bullet exit through the injured area. Since exit wounds are typically larger and more ragged than entry wounds, this might mask the underlying contusion. Maybe not, so you can have it either way.

Of course, the entry wound would need to be in such a location and the distance between the muzzle and the entry point would have to be short enough that the victim could have actually held the gun in that position and shot himself. For example, if the ME determined that the entry wound was a contact or nearly contact wound, was in the right temple, and the victim was right-handed (people almost always shoot themselves with the dominant hand), he might say that he could have done it himself. But if the wound is high and from behind and from a distance of more than two or three feet, he would conclude that the victim could not have done it. He would also check the victim's hands for gunshot residue, and if he found none would suspect that the victim had not fired the gun. Also, blood-spatter patterns on the floor, wall, and any objects in the area would have to match the victim's position at the time of the shooting, or the ME might suspect that the body was moved after the fact.

Your killer would have to take all this into account.

And if he moved the body he would also need to clean up the real crime scene and make sure that he left no drops of blood on the floor or furniture. If not, this type of evidence might do him in. In fact, it probably would. It is very difficult to stage a crime scene and fool investigators. Some tiny detail is almost always overlooked.

Is It Possible for the Coroner to Distinguish Between Murder and Suicide in a Hanging Victim?

Q: If my victim is found hanging by his belt, is there anyway the coroner can determine if it was a murder or a suicide?

A: The problem for the ME in this situation is not the cause and mechanism of death, but the manner. Let me explain.

The cause of death is the disease or injury that led to death. In this case it is hanging. The mechanism is the physiological abnormality that the cause of death produced that actually led to the death. In this case it is either asphyxia (death from lack of oxygen) or what is called spinal shock from a fractured neck and damaged spinal cord. In hangings the victim can die from either or both of these mechanisms.

If the drop is far enough, and if the belt holds, it will fracture the cervical vertebrae (neck bones) and damage the spinal cord. This shuts down the breathing center, which lies in the upper portion of the spinal cord, and also causes all the blood vessels of the body to relax, thus dropping the blood pressure to very low levels (spinal shock). The person dies instantly from a combination of asphyxia and shock.

If the drop does not fracture the neck, the belt serves as a ligature and strangles the victim. Here the death is from asphyxia, and is slower and more painful.

Now, to the manner of death, which is your question. There are four manners of death: natural, accidental, suicidal, and homicidal. A natural death can be ruled out in this case, since there is nothing natural about hanging.

An accidental death could be ruled if the ME felt that this was part of some autoerotic ritual that got out of hand, or some other accidental occurrence. For some reason the asphyxia of partial or near hanging makes sexual excitement more intense in some people. This can occur with solo or partner sexual activity.

That leaves suicidal and homicidal. The distinction is, who put the rope around the victim's neck: the victim or someone else. This may be very difficult to determine. Both suicidal and homicidal hangings can result in a fractured neck, with instant death, or in a slower death from strangulation, since the mechanism of death depends upon how effective the hanging is and not on who initiated the events.

Persons who die from strangulation/asphyxiation in a botched hanging often struggle and fight for survival. This is true even in suicide attempts, since once the rope tightens and the victim is still alive, he gets religion. What looked good on paper is not so attractive in reality. He would try to climb the rope, tug it from his neck, and claw at his throat. This leaves behind scratches and tears, and maybe a fingernail or two. Not pretty.

But these same struggles could occur regardless of who put the rope around the victim's neck. This means these findings do not distinguish between suicide and homicide. Neither do any of the typical findings at autopsy in a hanging death: ligature bruises of the neck; petechial hemorrhages (red dots and spots) of the conjunctivae (pink parts around the eyeball); and asphyxial changes in the lungs.

So, are there any specific findings that would suggest that the hanging was homicide? The presence of enough drugs in the victim's blood that would preclude his ability to do the deed, other injuries to the victim that he could not have inflicted upon himself, or the victim's hands tied behind his back would suggest homicide. One point about tied hands deserves mention. Just because the hands are tied does not mean the victim didn't commit suicide. Often people who choose this method will tie their own hands to prevent them from backing out at the last minute. The key is: Could the victim have tied the knots that bound his hands? Some knots can be self-tied, while others can't. The ME would consider this in making his determination. He might even call in a forensic knot expert. Yes, these individuals exist, and it is a fascinating art.

In your scenario, if you want the ME to believe this was a homicide, I'd have the ME find bruises on the victim that showed he had been restrained (bruises on the arms or signs of blows to the head), or find a high level of sedatives in his blood, which would mean he was too sedated to have hung himself. Or have his hands tied in such a fashion that the victim could not have done it.

Can the Examination of the Entrance Wound on a Murder Victim Show That the Weapon Used Had a Silencer?

Q: I have a question about handgun wounds. My victim is shot in the back of the head from a distance of about one to two feet. Is it possible to ascertain whether a silencer was used?

A: If you are talking about the character of the wound, the answer is, not likely. If you are talking about evaluating the bullet or test firing the suspect weapon, the answer is, maybe. Let me explain.

When a gun is fired the gunpowder explodes, forcing the bullet from the cartridge and down the gun's barrel. But the bullet is not the only thing that leaves the barrel. Hot gases and particulate matter are also ejected from the muzzle. The gases are predominantly carbon monoxide, carbon dioxide, and nitrogen oxide. Mixed with these gases are certain components of the primer. The most important of these are the heavy metals lead, bismuth, and antimony, which are useful when testing for gunshot residue. The particulate matter is burned and unburned powder, and soot.

Each of these ejected materials travels different distances from the muzzle. The hot gases may travel only a few inches, the particulate matter a foot or two, and, of course, the bullet a considerable distance. The character of the entry wound will depend upon which of these components actually contact the skin. The ME can use this information to determine the distance between the gun's muzzle and the point of entry at the moment the gun discharged.

The anatomy of the entrance wound depends upon how close the muzzle is to the skin. If two or more feet away, the entrance wound would be a small hole, smaller than the bullet, due to the elastic quality of skin. There would be a blue-black bruising effect in a halo around the entry point (called an "abrasion collar") and some black smudging where the skin literally wiped the bullet clean of the burned powder, grime, and oil residue it picked up as it passed through the barrel. This smudging is often easily wiped away with a wet cloth.

If the muzzle is between six inches and two feet from the point of entry, there might also be tattooing or stippling of the skin. This is due to burned and unburned powder that is discharged from the muzzle. These tiny particles imbed in the skin and/or cause tiny hemorrhages (red dots of blood within the skin) in a speckled pattern around the wound. These cannot be wiped off, because the particles are actually imbedded (tattooed) into the skin. The breadth of scatter or spread of this stippling increases as the distance between the muzzle and the entry point increases. The tattooing resulting from a gunshot inflicted from a distance of ten or twelve inches will be compact, and dense, while that from a shot delivered from eighteen to twenty-four inches will be broader and less dense.

If the muzzle is only a few inches away, the stippling will be very compact and partially obliterated by the charring from the hot gases. Here the skin around the entry wound is burned and blackened by the heat from the expelled gases. In addition, the carbon monoxide in the gases combines with hemoglobin and myoglobin (iron-containing compounds that reside in the blood and muscle tissues, respectively). This combination produces carboxyhemoglobin and carboxymyoglobin. These compounds are bright red in color and impart this to the surrounding tissues. Thus, a gunshot from a very close distance will produce a hole, a compact area of stippling, a surrounding area of charring, and a bright red hue to the wounded tissues.

A contact gunshot wound occurs when the gun's muzzle is pressed against the skin as it is fired. In this circumstance the hot gases and particulate matter are driven directly into the skin, producing greater charring. Also, the rapidly expanding gases rip the skin in a star-shaped, or stellate, pattern. Since the gases cannot expand the gun's metal barrel, nor can they force their way very deeply into the tissues, they take the path of least resistance by expanding laterally in every direction and tearing the skin in a jagged star pattern. This is particularly true if the contact wound is over a bone such as the skull. Thus, a contact wound will rip the skin in a classic stellate pattern, char the skin severely, and produce the bright red tissue color described above.

The presence of an extension such as a silencer may affect these patterns, but not in any predictable way. Let's say the muzzle was a few inches from the victim's skin. Whether the muzzle was the end of the barrel or the end of the silencer, the wound would look more or less the same. Unless the silencer was quite long. In this case, there may be much less charring, since the gases would have more time to cool before reaching the skin. Still, there are no reliable signs that would indicate that a silencer was used. With a couple of exceptions, that is.

If the silencer was packed with some sound-deadening material, fragments and fibers could be carried out with the gases and imbedded in the victim's skin. Silencers have also been made using steel wool, plastic milk bottles, towels, pillows, and all sorts of materials. If the ME saw fragments of any of these in the wound he might suggest that a silencer was used.

Also, an examination of the bullets removed from the victim might help determine that a silencer was used. This would require that the examiner have the suspect weapon and silencer for comparison. Let me explain. When the firearms examiner compares a crime-scene bullet with a test-fired bullet he looks at the grooves and striations that the rifled barrel carved into the sides of the bullets. If these match he will say that both bullets came from the same gun. If not, they came from different guns, and the gun in question is not the murder weapon.

If the silencer added any striations to the crime-scene bullet, and if the examiner test fired the suspect gun with the silencer in place, he might be able to match the two bullets and conclude that this gun with this silencer fired the killing bullet. If he only had one of these—the gun or the silencer, but not both—any test firing might not yield a match.

So either matching the bullet striations with the gun and the silencer, or finding extraneous materials in the wound that came from the silencer, might lead the ME to conclude that a silencer was indeed used by the killer.

Is It Possible That a Recent Blood Transfusion Could Confuse DNA Analysis?

Q: If a person has recently had a blood transfusion— within a few days of being killed—would their blood show two different types of DNA? I know eventually the recipient's body would replace all the transfused blood, but in the interim, what would the outcome be?

Debbie Bouchillon
Bartow, Florida

A: DNA testing is done on the DNA found in the nucleus of cells. Most cells in the body have nuclei, but the blood's red blood cells (RBCs) do not. Thus, they have no DNA. When blood is used for DNA sampling we are actually using the DNA in the white blood cells (WBCs).

If a person received a transfusion it is possible that a blood sample taken could reveal confusing results in DNA profiling for a few weeks. This is particularly true if several pints of blood had been given. Of course, each pint would likely come from a different donor, so actually, the patient would end up with WBCs from several people, and would thus possess several different types of nuclear DNA.

If the transfusion did interfere, and confusing DNA profiles resulted, which is possible, this could be rectified by taking cells from elsewhere, such as from the lining of the mouth. The transfused blood would not contaminate these cells. This process, called a buccal smear, is a simple process of gently scraping the inside of the cheek.

So, yes, a transfusion could confuse the results of DNA testing, and, yes, there are ways around it.

What Would the ME See Internally at Autopsy That Would Reveal Exactly What Surgical Procedures the Corpse Had Undergone?

Q: Is it possible to determine from an autopsy whether or not a person has undergone any internal surgical procedures? There would be external scars, of course, but would there be internal scarring that could tell the ME exactly what procedure had been done?

A: Most often yes. Most surgical procedures are to remove something (appendectomy, gallbladder removal, many cancer surgeries) or to repair something (coronary artery bypass, hernia repairs). In most cases the ME would be able to see what had been removed or repaired. Not always, since sometimes things aren't that easy. However, as you might guess, it is typically easier to determine that something is missing than it is to determine that something has been repaired.

If the surgery was recent, say two to four months, it would be very easy to see that a repair had been done. The scars would be fresher and more visible. But after ten years it might not be so easy. Scars tend to pale and shrink with time, and they might become virtually invisible. This takes years in most cases.

Part V

Odds and Ends—Mostly Odds

What Is the Cause of Death in a Crucifixion?

Q: I have a question about a historical manuscript that I am writing. What is the actual cause of death when someone is crucified?

Carla Fanning
Granada Hills, California

A: The cause of death is hypovolemic shock with cardiac arrest and hypoxia from compromise of the lungs. Let's look at shock first.

"Hypo" means low; "volemia" means volume of fluid within the vascular system; and "shock" means the blood pressure (BP) is lowered to the point that the tissues of the body are not receiving enough oxygen (O_2) and nutrients. Cardiac arrest is when the heart stops, or at least is no longer effective as a pump to move the blood around the body.

The cardiovascular system is a closed system, which means that all the blood remains within the confines of the heart and the blood vessels. The pressure within the system (the blood pressure, or BP) is determined by many factors, with one of the most important being how full the system is. With loss of blood or with extreme dehydration from excessive sweating, the volume within the system drops (hypovolemia), and so does the BP. Another way to decrease the pressure is to expand the volume of the system while keeping the amount of blood the same.

An analogy would be a car tire. If air is bled out, the pressure within the tire will drop. If the amount of air is kept the same, while the size (volume) of the tire is increased, the pressure inside will drop. So, to lower the pressure in any closed system you either remove some of the contents or expand the size of the system.

The blood vessels of the body have great capacity to constrict (clamp down) and dilate (open up). This allows for the distribution of blood to where it is needed. Whenever you stand up, the veins of the legs constrict to prevent gravity-induced pooling of the blood in the legs. If this pooling were allowed to occur, the amount of blood available for the brain would be reduced. This constriction of the veins happens automatically all day, every day. In some people this reflex is defective, and they have what we call orthostatic or positional dizziness. When these people stand, the reflex constriction of the leg veins does not occur, blood pools in the legs, blood to the brain is diminished, and the person becomes dizzy, and may even pass out. This is very common in military recruits who stand at attention in the hot sun. The constriction mechanism in the veins fatigues and fails, allowing blood to drop into the legs, and dizziness and loss of consciousness follows. The recruit awakens upon hitting the ground, when gravity now allows blood to move back toward the brain. The dehydration and hypovolemia that occur from standing in the sun makes this more likely. In this case the volume of fluid within the closed system drops, and the size of the system increases (with the loss of constriction of the veins). These two events work together to drop the BP and lead to fainting.

A crucifixion is similar. The victim is nailed to a cross, usually in an area exposed to the sun. He sweats into hypovolemia, the BP falls, and he faints. This may take several hours. But unlike the military recruits, he cannot fall, so gravity remains his enemy. The blood continues to pool in the legs, and the supply to the brain and heart continues to decline until brain death and/or a cardiac arrest lead to death. To hasten the death the victim is often lanced in the side. The bleeding that results from this adds to the hypovolemia from the sweating, thus bringing about death more quickly.

Another factor in crucifixion is a crushing of the lungs. As the victim becomes weaker from low BP and fatigue, his shoulders will sag and his body will collapse forward. This will compress the chest and, in effect, crush the lungs. As this crushing progresses the lungs will no longer function effectively, and the oxygen content in the blood will begin to fall. This will conspire with the shock mentioned above and bring about death.

This is a slow and painful process.

Could My Character Hide Inside a Corpse?

Q: I'm considering an odd idea for a horror story. My character is a small woman who must protect herself from a cold environment. If she were to open the corpse of a man and crawl inside, what would she need to remove? She's very small and he is a large man. And once this is done, how long does the human body stay warm after death? Is it possible for her to stay warm inside a dead body for four to five hours? Would this even work?

Tiffany Tripp
Costa Mesa, California

A: This is an extremely clever and diabolical idea. I love it.

The smaller the woman and the bigger the man, the more likely this is to work. Regardless, she would need to empty the corpse completely. She would open the abdomen from the base of the breastbone to the pubic area. This would leave the ribs intact so that her hiding place would be more structurally sound. If the ribs were removed, which is a very difficult proposition, the body would simply collapse.

She would empty the abdomen. Bladder, kidneys, intestines, stomach, liver, pancreas, and spleen would all be removed. She could then remove the diaphragm, and reach into the chest and remove the heart, lungs, and esophagus. After this she would have a completely empty corpse and could curl herself into the remaining cavity.

A body cools at about 1.5 degrees per hour, but after the removal of the internal organs it would cool more rapidly. Regardless, it will only drop to the ambient temperature. If the corpse is in a room, it would gradually drop to room temperature. If out in the cold, it would drop to the air temperature surrounding the body. If in a hot garage in August in Houston, the corpse might actually gain temperature.

If she is in an exposed and very cold area this would protect her the way a small ice cave would, which can be life saving when stranded in a snowstorm. The ice cave captures body heat and keeps it from escaping into the air, and it also protects the person from the wind and cold. A hollowed-out corpse would work the same way for your young lady, and she could easily survive for the four or five hours you need.

How Long After Immersion Would a Head Found in a Wooden Box in the North Sea Still Be Recognizable?

Q: I'm writing a novel set in Roman Britain in A.D. 90. Can you please tell me how quickly a severed head would decay in the North Sea? It is washed ashore in a wooden chest, so no fish have gotten to it. Since my sleuth needs to recognize the head, I need to know what the longest time is that a head could remain in the sea and still be identifiable, assuming it was freshly dead when it was put in the chest and the voyage lasted only two or three days before the shipwreck?

A: If the head sat in the box for two or three days before the ship sank and dumped it into the water, it would decompose more rapidly than if the head had been severed and placed into the box just before the ship went down. Decay of human tissues is due to bacteria. On board the head would be relatively warm, and this favors bacterial growth, and thus putrefaction (decay).

The North Sea, on the other hand, is more hostile to bacteria. The cold alone would delay decay, and the salinity (salt content) would also serve as an antibacterial. Most bacteria do not thrive in cold and salty environments. The box would at least partially fill with the cold water, unless it were completely airtight, which would be unlikely in the time period of your story.

So, if the head lay around for several days before going into the sea, the decay process would be well under way by the time it landed in the water. The bacteria would already have done some destruction, and it would have a "foothold." This would lead to a more rapid deterioration. It would be like leaving meat out for a day, and then placing it into the refrigerator. It would decay faster than meat that was refrigerated from the beginning, but slower than any left out indefinitely. If this is your scenario, I would not extend the time beyond one to two weeks.

If the head found itself in the cold water immediately after the severing, no bacterial "foothold" and decay would occur; once the head was in the cold water the decay process would be greatly delayed. This is like placing the meat directly into the refrigerator. Here, three to four, or even as much as eight, weeks before the head washed ashore would not be unreasonable.

Of course, in both scenarios the facial tissues would swell and deform, but less so in the latter. If the victim had some unusual facial characteristic such as a hawkish nose, broad ears, wide-set eyes, or a scar, the identification would be easier.

The bottom line is that the sooner the head is dropped into the cold water after its removal, and the sooner it washes to shore and is found, the better.

How Long Does It Take for a Laxative to Take Effect?

Q: My character doesn't want to kill his victims, just cause a heck of a lot of discomfort. He plans to add chocolate Ex-Lax or a similar product to baked goods, and then feed them to his victims. My timeline requires that symptoms begin to occur within an hour or two of ingestion. Is this feasible? And what would be the most common side effects other than the most obvious?

A: Send me your number. I want to talk with your mother.

Laxatives come in many varieties and work by different mechanisms. Some lubricate (mineral oil), some add bulk and water (Metamucil and fiber-containing products), some draw water into the colon and form liquid stools (magnesium citrate), and some stimulate the colon to contract (Ex-Lax). None of these are absorbed into the body, so they have no toxic effects on the body as a whole. This means you don't have to worry about killing your characters with laxatives.

So Ex-Lax would work well for your purposes. Depending upon how much is given, the size and weight of the person, what his or her normal diet is, and other factors, the time until the victim knows something is going on could be in the range of thirty minutes to two hours or so. Shortly thereafter the victims would need to trot off to the nearest restroom, thus the origin of the phrase "the trots."

This broad range means that you can construct your plot as you need. Have the effects occur somewhere between twenty minutes and two hours, and you'll be okay.

Can My Character Die from an Imagined Disease?

Q: What is the correct terminology for injuries resulting from imaginary or psychosomatic insults to the body, such as those outbreaks of rashes and asthma caused by a fear reaction to a nontoxic gas release? How severe can these be? Can someone actually die from "choking" on a nontoxic gas that they believed to be toxic?

Soni Pitts
Poplar Bluff, Missouri

A: The general terms used are "psychogenic," which means the symptoms are generated in the psyche, and "hypochondriacal," which means illnesses imagined where none are present.

Hives (a blisterlike rash) and asthmalike symptoms can definitely occur with psychogenic stressors, but they typically feel and appear to an untrained observer more severe than they are. That said, yes, people can die from extreme psychological stress and panic. This type of stress can cause a massive outpouring of adrenaline from the adrenal glands, which lie within the abdomen near the kidneys. This large output of adrenaline can cause deadly cardiac arrhythmias (changes in heart rhythm) and spasm (clamping down and narrowing) of the coronary arteries that can lead to a myocardial infarction (MI, or heart attack). This would be particularly true if the victim had underlying coronary artery disease (hardening of the arteries) in the first place.

Your panicked victim would develop shortness of breath, a rapid and heavy heartbeat, chest pain, maybe wheezing and a rash, and could then collapse and die.

What Happens When You "Get the Wind Knocked Out of You"?

Q: What happens when you "get the wind knocked out of you"? I have a character in my short story who suffers a blow to his midsection, and this happens to him.

A: This occurs with a strong blow to the pit of the stomach. There is a collection of nerves in that area, deep behind the stomach, called the solar plexus. A blow to this area can cause a massive outpouring of impulses, which in turn will cause the diaphragm to spasm (cramp). While this is happening the diaphragm is frozen, so breathing isn't possible. After a few seconds, or up to a minute, the diaphragm relaxes and breathing is once again possible. Scary and painful, but not deadly.

Do Zombie Killers Leave Behind Forensic Evidence?

Q: What kind of physical or forensic evidence would be left behind if the murderer were actually a dead woman? Yes, this is a supernatural novel, so I get to fudge all kinds of things, but I want it to be mostly accurate. Would my zombielike dead killer's hair, skin, body fluids, fingerprints, etc., be identifiable to investigators as belonging to someone who is dead?

Carla Jablonski

New York, New York

Author of *Thicker Than Water* and other novels

A: Since you're dealing with a zombie anything is possible, and you can have it any way you want. Sci-fi and horror have few rules. For sure, hair and fingerprints would be just the same as they would be in a living person. Hair is basically dead anyway, and fingerprints are just patterned smudges left by the oils and dirt that collect on the finger pads. This would be the same whether the person was dead or alive.

As for blood, body fluids, and hair follicles, it depends upon whether your zombies have normal tissues and normal blood, and whether they bleed or not. You can make their blood and tissues appear normal or abnormal as you need for your plot. If abnormal they might have odd-looking or abnormal cells, or they might have unusual proteins in their blood.

Your killer could leave behind some hair with the follicles attached, or some blood. Analysis could show that it was normal in every way or not. If not, the red and white cells within the blood could appear odd. Perhaps too large or too small or too irregular in shape. Your investigators could find abnormal proteins within the blood plasma or the tissues. The zombie DNA could be very different from normal. Finding any of these abnormalities would tip off your sleuth that the killer wasn't one of us. Dum-duh-da-dum.

Can My ME Determine That a Character Was Killed by a Boa Constrictor?

Q: If a boa constrictor is used as a murder weapon, what exactly would be the cause of death, and would my ME be able to determine that?

Gay Toltl Kinman
Alhambra, California
Author of *Castle Reiner* and *Super Sleuth: Five Alison Leigh
Powers Mysteries*
gaykinman.com

A: Death in this situation would be from mechanical asphyxia, which results when some external force is applied to the body that prevents the expansion of the chest, and thus respiration. A person trapped beneath a heavy object such as a car or a collapsed wall or ceiling may die from this. A similar circumstance occurs when people are crushed during a riot or trampled by a stampeding crowd. Think English soccer fans. In this situation the external pressure is so great that the victim literally can't take a breath.

A boa constrictor kills exactly this way. This muscular species of snake wraps itself around its prey. With each exhalation of the prey, the snake coils a little tighter. Thus, each successive breath becomes increasingly shallower, until the prey is trapped in the position of exhalation and is unable to take another breath. Death follows quickly.

Would the ME see any signs of this at autopsy? Maybe, maybe not. The victim could have petechial hemorrhages (small red dots or splotches) in the conjunctivae of the eye (the pink part around the eyeball). These are caused by blood leaking from the tiny capillaries of the conjunctivae due to the extreme pressure applied to the chest. He may also find bruises on the victim's arms, chest, back, and abdomen, and perhaps a few fractured ribs. Or he may find none of this, and the cause of death may not be identifiable.

Would a Corpse Decay on Mars?

Q: I am working on a screenplay where human remains are found on Mars. I am interested in what body decomposition would be like in an environment that is high in carbon dioxide and void of any bacteria. Would the body be mummified? Would it be similar to bodies found in the bogs of Europe? I'm guessing that decay would be minimal and the body would be intact.

A: Great question. Obviously no one knows for sure, since this circumstance has never occurred, but a review of known data from our unmanned Martian missions offers many possibilities.

In general bodies decompose by either putrefaction (decay) or mummification. Warm, damp environments favor bacterial growth and decay, while colder, drier climes favor mummification. Mummification might also occur in very hot and dry areas. Just like beef jerky, which is made in a hot, dry oven. The bacteria that are responsible for putrefaction mostly come from within the gastrointestinal tract of the corpse and not from the environment, so the fact that Mars has no bacteria, as far as we know, is not really an issue. The corpse would have plenty of its own.

By far the most important factor in whether bacteria grow or not is the ambient temperature. The data on Martian temperatures comes form the two Viking Landers, the Pathfinder mission, and the Viking Orbiter Infrared Thermal Mapper. Since Mars possesses a very thin atmosphere, temperature is predominately a reflection of solar heating and not wind and other weather. As is usual in such circumstances, Mars shows wide variations and fluctuations in surface temperatures. The average surface temperature on Mars is −63 degrees Fahrenheit, with a maximum of 68 degrees Fahrenheit and a minimum of −220. The Viking Orbiter found that temperatures may reach as low as −225 degrees Fahrenheit at the polar regions and as high as 81 degrees Fahrenheit in areas directly impacted by the sun's rays, usually toward the equator of the planet.

Most likely the corpse in your story would be frozen and perfectly preserved. This would be true particularly if it is near one of the polar regions or in a low-lying area shaded from direct sunlight. If the body were in an open area and exposed to direct sunlight for periods of each day, the temperature of at least the surface of the corpse could be such that the bacteria would grow and lead to some degree of decay. Remember that even in these circumstances, the corpse would remain frozen for most of the time, particularly inside. The nighttime temps would be well below zero, and the time of sun exposure would be only a few hours each day. It would take more than a few hours to thaw out the interior of a corpse that was frozen to a temperature of say −50 to −100 degrees Fahrenheit (the outer inch or so, but not the inside). This means that the body would decay somewhat on the surface, but the internal organs would be spared and remain preserved.

On Earth bodies decay from the inside (where the bacteria are located) out. But bodies found in snowy mountain regions that are exposed to direct sunlight during the day may show this outside-in pattern of decay, with relative sparing of the interior of the corpse. The same would likely happen on Mars, except that the overnight temps would be much, much lower, so the interior of the corpse would never thaw and would be perfectly preserved. One other factor is that in such scenarios, the bacteria that cause the surface decay tend to come from the environment, since the GI tract and its bacterial contents remain frozen. On Mars there would be no such bacteria, so even in direct sunlight the corpse might not decay at all. No one knows.

Bottom line is that your corpse would likely be frozen and would show no signs of decay. It may or may not show signs of thawing over the surface (if in an exposed area), and it is at least possible that it could show signs of some surface decay.

Since there is no known moisture on Mars, the body would gradually desiccate (dry out), making mummification a distinct possibility. So you can have it either way. Your corpse could be frozen and preserved, or could dehydrate and mummify. Or it could do a little of both.

Could the ME Determine That My Character Had Been Eaten by a Werewolf?

Q: I am writing a horror story about werewolves, and am going on the assumption that werewolf bites would be about twice the size of a normal wolf's. My victim runs into a wolflike creature that proceeds to eat him alive. I am wondering what the wounds would look like. Could the animal remove bone in one clean bite, or would it have to gnaw, and slowly eat it away? Would a medical examiner normally assume in this situation that it was a wolf or a bobcat, or would he look for another animal as the culprit?

John T. Eaton
Nashville, Tennessee

A: Either a werewolf or a real wolf would have no problem devouring muscles, tissues, and internal organs. A real wolf would likely have to gnaw away at the bones, but a werewolf has superhuman strength and could bite right through most bones. Or not. It's fiction, so do it any way you want.

The ME would examine the wounds and determine that they were a combination of punctures and slashes and might be able to measure them for depth, width, and, in the case of the punctures, the general shape of the weapon. In this case the puncture wounds would indicate that the weapon was a round, curved, pointed object like a fang. Also, there might be gnaw marks on the bones. From this information he could conclude that the attacker was a wolf or some other animal with large fangs. A bobcat is too small for consideration, but wolves, bears, and mountain lions could be responsible. And, of course, so could werewolves.

The ME wouldn't likely consider a werewolf as the killer. But he could find some hair or blood from the werewolf, and when he examined it microscopically and analyzed its DNA he would discover that it did not match that of any known species. Now he has a problem. What kind of animal did this? Until he actually found a werewolf and made comparisons between the victim's wounds and the werewolf's teeth, he could not say exactly what type of creature did the deed.

Can My Villain, Who Is Shot in the Head Just as He Is Being Teleported to Another Site, Survive the Gunshot?

Q: I am writing a science fiction short story that concludes with the hero shooting the villain during the final scene. However, the villain teleports himself the instant the bullet begins traveling through his brain. The timing between the bullet entering the villain's skull and his disappearance are so close that witnesses cannot immediately tell if he is hit or not. In fact, many wonder if the villain has escaped to another place, to continue his meddling with society.

I was wondering what evidence would be left behind. I plan to have the bullet continue on its path and hit the wall, but would there also be blood spatter and bits of brain? I'm not sure at what point during the bullet's flight the villain will teleport, but after the initial shock of the villain's disappearance, I want it to be evident fairly quickly to the hero that the villain is either dead or will die from his wounds.

This might be a question with an obvious answer, but are most shots to the head fatal?

Jason Schifano
Clifton, New Jersey

A: I hope I understand what you want, but I'm not entirely sure. It appears that in the world you have created, the transporter machine would only beam away the person and not the bullet, regardless of whether the bullet is still in the person or not. Further, it seems that if the bullet blows away any tissues from the person, those tissues would then remain behind with the bullet and would not be transported as well. And it appears that the scene continues at the site of the gunshot where the bullet remains and does not follow the victim to wherever he has been transported. I hope these assumptions are correct.

If so, the answer to your question is quite simple. If the bullet remains within the victim at the time of transport, only the bullet will be left. It could have some blood on it or not. That would depend upon the rules you have set for your transport device. If it would transport all living tissue within the person being transported, then even the tiniest drops of blood on the bullet would also be carried away. Or if it doesn't take everything down the transport path, blood could be left behind on the bullet. Minor point, but I'm not sure if your plot needs blood on the bullet or not. You can have it either way as long as your transport rules are consistent throughout the story. The point here is that a little blood on the bullet would not prove that the villain was dead, only injured. And no blood at all might indicate that the bullet had missed him entirely.

If the bullet exits the victim's head, then tissue and blood would be carried out through the exit wound and would spatter on the walls, floor, furniture, or anything nearby. If this is the case, our hero would assume that with the amount of blood and brain tissue left behind, the villain would certainly be dead.

Now, if you follow the victim to where he went, he would either have a hole in his head, the depth of which would be the depth the bullet had traveled at the time of transport, or if the bullet exited his head, he would have a gaping exit wound at that site and would likely be dead. Maybe not.

No, all gunshots to the head are not fatal. They can be as simple as flesh wounds, as deadly as the destruction of most of the brain, and anywhere in between.

What Is a Picarist?

Q: I am writing about a serial killer whose fetish is cutting his victims in a delicate, sexually deviant manner. I believe these types of deviants are called "picarists." Is this the correct term?

Katie McLaughlin
Santa Maria, California

A: The term "picarist" comes from the Latin and Spanish verb *picar*, which means "to prick" or "to perforate." The adjectives *pícaro* and *picarón* come from this root, and mean mischievous, wicked, sly, or impish. The actual term for the psychosexual disorder you describe is "piquerism," and those who practice this form of psychopathology are called "piquerists." However, I have seen both terms used. Regardless of what they are called, they are very bad characters.

A piquerist (or picarist) is someone who derives sexual gratification from torturing his victims with multiple tiny cuts, pricks, and stabs over a period of time.

Could My Bad Guy Be Severely Burned in a Tanning Bed?

Q: I have a bad guy trapped in a tanning bed. I want him to suffer much more than a sunburn, but don't want to kill him. Any ideas?

David Skibbins
The Sea Ranch, California
Author of *Eight of Swords* and *High Priestess*
www.davidskibbins.com

A: Ouch! This would do the trick.

Burns are of three degrees. First is like a severe sunburn, and usually heals without much treatment and without any complications.

Second is blistering and damage to the upper layers of the skin. This will heal and leave little if any scarring. It can become infected, and this can move it to a third-degree situation, since the infection will damage the deeper layers of the skin, and can even cause death from a blood infection (called septicemia, or sepsis).

Third-degree burns involve the deeper layers of the skin, lead to severe scarring, and require skin grafting to repair. This is very dangerous, and when these types of burns cover more than 50 percent of the body it carries a high mortality rate, usually from secondary infections. If the burns cover 90 percent of the body the mortality rate is over 90 percent.

In most burns there are areas of burning at each of these degrees.

How severely your guy gets burned depends upon how much of his skin is exposed, the length of the exposure, and the level of UV radiation the particular unit puts out. The units used in tanning booths are not uniform. I'd guess that five to ten minutes would do a good first; ten to fifteen minutes a second; and fifteen or more would be big trouble for the guy. These are very ballpark guesses, but in the context of fiction they would work.

How Could My Sleuth Recognize a Chimera?

Q: My question is about chimeras, individuals whose bodies are made up of two genetically different lines of cells. The case I read about involved a woman who underwent tests to determine if one of her sons was suitable as a kidney donor for her. Testing determined that two of her sons were *not* her biological children. Their DNA came from the mother's twin, who instead of surviving to be born was somehow absorbed into the birth mother's body.

I would love to use this as a springboard for fiction, but I need some help to be sure I'm on at least semisolid ground. Unless the character with this condition needed an organ transplant, would there be any other possible way for the condition to be diagnosed?

Susanne Shaphren
Phoenix, Arizona
Author of "Arrangements," in *Mystery Writers of America
Presents Show Business Is Murder,* and "The Best of
Friends," in *Sex, Lies, & Private Eyes*

A: When an egg and a sperm join to make a fertilized egg, the genetic makeup of the offspring is set at that moment. Normally the cell will divide into two, and those into four, and those into eight, and so on. At some point in the growth of the zygote the cells begin to specialize, or what we call "differentiate." Some will become brain tissue, others blood cells, and others muscle cells.

In fraternal twins two eggs are fertilized by two sperm, and this process occurs in parallel, and two entirely distinct individuals result. In identical twins the original fertilized cell (egg) divides into two cells, but these two drift apart, and then each proceeds along the growth path in tandem. This creates two individuals with identical genetics. After all, they started from the same cell, and thus from the same egg and sperm. So far so good.

In chimeras fraternal twins are formed (two eggs and two sperm, and two genetically different individuals), but these two original cells (fertilized eggs) stick together. As growth takes place the developing zygote is composed of two distinctively different cell types with two distinctively different genetic makeups. As these cells begin to specialize, some organs and tissues may come from one type of cell and some from the other, and still others may develop with a mixture of cell types. This leads to a chimera, where various body tissues (liver, blood, skin, heart, brain) may have one or the other or both of the two original DNA profiles. This can lead to confusion in any testing dependent upon DNA typing.

Chimeras may appear normal or may display certain mosaic patterns, particularly unusual pigmentation patterns, on their skin. This is merely an expression of their two genetic types. A mosaic in art is something made up of different-appearing distinct pieces. The same holds true here, since the cells of the person contain separate and distinctive DNA patterns.

If the person were normal in appearance, the only time a chimeric condition would be diagnosed would be if DNA testing were undertaken. This is done in organ transplantation, paternity testing, and in criminal situations, to name a few circumstances. Otherwise the person may never know of his condition.

If your character displayed an odd mosaic skin pattern, your sleuth could see this and suspect that the person was chimeric. These skin patterns can be almost anything, even areas of a distinct checkerboard pattern.

How Could Shakespeare's Titus Grind Two Corpses Fine Enough to Use in a Minced Pie?

Q: I am writing a paper about Shakespeare's *Titus Androni-cus*. At the end of the play, Titus takes the two sons of Tamora and cuts them into little pieces, grinds them up, and makes minced pie from them. My question is: What would that labor have entailed? How difficult would that have been?

A: I believe it was Mark Twain who said something like, "A man has no need to know how laws or frankfurters are made." Your sce-nario is similar to sausage or hotdog making.

Titus would not have modern-day grinders, or even the hand-cranked ones of the more recent past. This means that his work would be long and arduous. His tools would be a knife, a saw, and an axe. The first thing you need to determine is: Did he grind up the entire body (including the bones) or just the flesh and organs?

I'll assume he used the muscles and organs and discarded the bones, since these, even if finely chopped, would be detectable in the pies. He might use a mortar and pestle to grind the bones to a fine powder and use it, but this would be a tremendous amount of work.

First he would hack and saw off the arms, legs, and head. Each section would then be dealt with separately. He would use the knife to strip off the skin and cut away the meat and remove all the internal organs. The axe would open the skull. He would then simply keep cutting and chopping the tissues, muscles, and organs until they reached the size he desired. This would take hours and would be very exhausting. He would fight fatigue and cramping in his hands and forearms unless he were a manual laborer such as a blacksmith. The average person would find this an extremely diffi-cult task.

If he had access to a large stone grain mill, his task would be eas-ier. He could simply section up the body and place it between the stones and kick-start the mules or whatever animal served as its power source. Of course, these old stone grinders were very crude and the bones would be chunked but not finely ground, and would thus be noticeable.

Would Abraham Lincoln Have Survived His Injuries Today?

Q: This is a pure curiosity question. Do you think that Lincoln could have been saved if they had today's medical knowledge, techniques, and equipment in 1864?

Martha Kuhn
Mt. Gilead, Ohio

A: Most likely, yes. He was shot in the back of his head, and the bullet apparently entered his brain. He lived for many hours, so the shot was not immediately fatal. A surgeon probed the wound but feared removing the bullet, since it might have caused bleeding. He probably should have, but we'll never know.

Similar wounds today are treated by a trip to the OR, removal of the bullet, controlling bleeding, and preventing any subsequent infection. He would have had at least a 50 percent chance of survival. And since he survived several hours anyway, the likelihood of his survival with modern techniques would be much higher.

Could My Character Choke to Death on a Scarf She Used to Fake the Regurgitation of Ectoplasm?

Q: I'm killing off a character who is attempting to fool others into believing that she is regurgitating ectoplasm, when in fact she is using a piece of muslin. I want her to choke on the material and die. That's the theory, anyway. It's based on what I've read about early mediums regurgitating materials to produce this effect, and that people can choke while vomiting. Is this at all plausible? What would the body look like shortly after death?

A: Yes, this could work easily.

The cloth could easily become wadded in her throat as she attempted to regurgitate it. This would block her airway and prevent air from reaching the lungs. She would become terrified and short of breath, and would struggle to breathe, and might even claw at her neck and mouth in an attempt to draw in air. She would become weaker, her struggles would lessen, and she would finally lapse into unconsciousness and die. This could take anywhere from about one to three minutes if the airway was completely obstructed and longer if only partially so, since she would be able to draw in a little air in this situation. Not enough to live but enough to prolong her death.

As she struggled she would deplete the oxygen (O_2) in her blood rapidly, and since it could not be replenished, she would become rapidly hypoxic (have a low oxygen level in the blood). As the O_2 level dropped she would become cyanotic. This is a manifestation of the bluish color of blood that has a low O_2 content. It gives the skin a blue-gray color, which is most prominent in the face, hands, and feet, since these areas tend to show cyanosis more prominently than the trunk of the body.

Immediately after death she would appear pale, waxy, and with cyanosis of her face, hands, and feet. The entire corpse could be slightly cyanotic, but the face, hands, and feet would be more so. She could also have scratch marks on her throat and around her mouth where she clawed herself in an attempt to get air. Lastly, she could have petechial hemorrhages (small red dots or splotches) in the conjunctivae (pink parts around the eyeball). These are due to blood leaking from the tiny capillaries in that area, which would result from the increased pressure in the blood vessels of her neck and head as she violently struggled to breathe.

A FEW FINAL WORDS

Now that you have completed this book, I hope you have learned something from the questions and answers inside. Some questions were simple and straightforward; others complex, sophisticated; and still others downright bizarre.

Yet, each question reveals the incredible imagination, curiosity, and dedication to getting it right that is essential for credible story-telling and fiction writing. As I said in the introduction, I believe these questions provide insight into the creative process and demonstrate the depth of commitment to craft that is found in successful writers of fiction.

I hope you found these pages interesting, informative, and stimulating. It is my sincerest wish that this information will improve your own writing and reading, and will stir your creative juices.

Thank you for your time, interest, and curiosity.

Visit Dr. Lyle's Web site, the Writer's Medical and Forensics Lab, at www.dplylemd.com.

INDEX